DICTIONARY OF
FILMS AND FILM TECHNOLOGY

DICTIONARY OF FILMS AND FILM TECHNOLOGY

By

Gangadhar Mahambare

ANMOL PUBLICATIONS PVT. LTD.
NEW DELHI - 110 002 (INDIA)

ANMOL PUBLICATIONS PVT. LTD.
4374/4B, Ansari Road, Daryaganj
New Delhi - 110 002
www.anmolbooks.com

Dictionary of Films and Film Technology

First Edition, 2002

ISBN 81-261-1027-9

PRINTED IN INDIA

Published by J.L. Kumar for Anmol Publications Pvt. Ltd., New Delhi - 110 002 and Printed at Mehra Offset Press, Delhi.

OUR TRIBUTE TO SRI SATYAJIT RAY

It was the earnest desire of film-maker Mr. Satyajit Ray that Mr. Gangadhar Mahambare should take up the task of compiling 'Dictionary of Films'. In this context Mr. Ray had replied to him either by correspondence or/and in person at Ray's residence in Calcutta. Mr. Mahambare's book on 'Oscar-award Winner Satyajit Ray was published in 1992 during the life-time of Mr. Ray.

This Dictionary is dedicated to Mr. Ray.

Preface

This Dictionary has been compiled to cover terminology pertaining to Films and Filming. These terms have been carefully selected and most of these are in vogue in the film industry that is spread world-over. This Dictionary also includes terms from the films' allied fields such as television, video etc.

Throughout the preparation of this edition of the Dictionary, the guiding principle has been to make it useful to all those who are basically interested in this subject.

In compiling a Dictionary of this kind of a subject, it becomes necessary to draw upon the work of many authorities. I am thankful to all those stalwarts who have made it possible to compile the Dictionary in the present form. I do not wish to claim any credit. However, I would like to mention here that I have deep interest in the subject both in principle and in practice. I have had the privilege to work as the First Librarian of the then Film Institute, Pune in early 1960s. My Marathi book entitled *'Life of Phalke—Father of the Indian Films'* has been added to the Library of Congress, Washington DC. Besides, I have written lyrics for few Marathi films and was declared as a winner for script writing in one of the Government of India's competition. I have also in the past prepared a 'Market Survey of Indian

Films'—the project which was assigned to me by M/s Impexport, Canada.

Lastly, I am thankful to the entire staff of Anmol Publications Pvt. Ltd., New Delhi, who have shown their keen interest in my work.

Readers are requested to feel free in expressing their comments and suggestions which will enable us to consider these while publishing the next edition.

'Shivaranjani'
12, Kalanagar, Pune-411043 **—Gangadhar Mahambare**
(India)

A

'AA' Certificate. Film category introduced by the British Board of Film Censors (BBFC) in 1970. The certificate describes that parents might consider the film for their children.

Abby Singer Shot. The second-to-last shot of the day. Named after Abby Singer, as assistant director, who worked for the Universal Studio and who would frequently call 'last shot of the day' only to have the director ask for one more take.

Above-the-line costs. In films, expenses pertaining the cast, director, producer and story.

Academy. Start mark appearing twelve feet before the first frame of the picture.

Academy cinema. The Institute founded by Elise Cohen in London in 1931, with the object of showing interesting films to natives.

Academy frame. A frame-size standardized by the Academy of Motion Picture of Arts & Sciences.

Academy of Motion Picture of Arts & Sciences (AMPAS). The Academy formed by the United States Film Industry in 1927 with the declared aim of raising the educational, cultural and technical standards of film-making. AMPAS owns a collection of films and an extensive library of printed matter relating to films. It presents annually Oscar awards for outstanding achievement in the previous years productions. The term 'Oscar' was coined by a lady film-journalist who spontaneously on seeing the statue remarked that the statue looked like her Uncle Oscar. (Very often wrongly ascribed to Oscar Wilde's (Irish Playwright's) name.

Academy of Motion Picture Sound. (AMPS). Academy formed in United States with the declared aim of promoting and encouraging the science, technology and creative application of all aspects of motion picture, sound recording and reproduction, and to promote and enhance the status and recognition of the contribution of those engaged therein.

Accelerando. (In music) A gradual change of meter f. om a slower to a faster tempo.

Acceptance angle. The area of view that falls within the sight lines of a lens or photosensitive cell.

Action. During filming 'action' is called to indicate the start of the proposed current take. The vital point of attention within each frame.

Action car. Vehicle in which actors ride as part of a scene during a moving car shot.

Actor/Actress. A person who plays the role of a character in a film or for that matter in any performing art. Now-a-days a term actor is referred for both genders.

Actu?lite. A documentary-type film known from the earliest work by the Lumiere Brothers in France.

Adaptation. A script of the film (or drama/TV play) in which suitable subject matter is translated for filming.

Additional camera. (B Camera). An extra camera operator often needed for complicated action sequences or stunts of filming. (Contrast with additional film-photography).

Additional photography. (Addl. photographer, Pickups, Reshoots, Reshooting). Studio reaction of having some shots or scenes are bad enough to convince the film-makers to discard them. In some cases, actors are therefore recalled for shooting purposes and parts of the movie are refilmed.

Additive process. A system of colour photography that adds together lights of the three additive primary colours i.e. red, green and blue in different degrees to form an image.

Advance. (In monetary terms). An amount given before receipt of the services. (In composite print) The distance between a point on the sound track and the corresponding image.

Agent. A professional manager, who deals with actor, director, music director and/or other artists. Very many times an agent negotiates the contracts on behalf of his clients viz. actor, director etc. In western countries an agent selects or recommends roles for their client.

Agfa Colour. A system developed by Agfa-filmfabrik in 1996.

Aleatory technique. The use of chance conditions and probability found in documentary direct cinema.

Althescope. A large single lens used in looking at transparency or an ordinary positive.

Ambient sound. The general background sound to any shooting situation, without which the dialogue or other specific sound seems to exist in a vacuum.

American Film Institute. (AFI). Founded in June 1967 with funds from American Government and the three reputed Organisations viz. Ford Foundation, National Foundation for the Arts and The Motion Picture of American Association (MPAA). AFI is located at JF Kennedy Centre for the Performing Arts in Washington D.C.

American Society of Cinematographers. (ASC). The Society was founded with the object of advancing the art of cinematography through artistry and technological progress in the profession. It interacts with the cinematographers on various aspects of cinematography. On getting recommendation by an existing member society provides membership to new professional entrants. The society is bringing out its official publication entitled 'American Cinematographer' regularly.

Amperage. (In electricity). Strength (value) of electrical current flowing through a circuit.

Anamorphic. (Cinemascope). An optical system which has different magnifications in the horizontal and vertical dimensions of the picture. Cinemascope has been given as a tradename to the anamorphic technique.

Anamorphic lens. Lens containing a cylindrical element.

Angle on. A camera term indicating that the angle should be on the person or thing but not specifying a focal length, such as medium close-up or close-up.

Angle shot. A shot continuing the action of a preceding shot, but from a different angle.

Animation. (Animated, Animator). The process of creating illusion of motion by creating individual frames, as opposed to filming naturally occurring action at a regular frame rate. Apparent movement of inanimate objects or drawings.

Anime. A peculiar style of animated movie. This style has its roots in the comic books of Japan. Since variety of subjects are covered in Anime this style has gained popularity among Japanese audiences. 'Anime' is very often used to describe exclusively the adult-oriented science fiction outside of Japan. Fantasy entries in the field are also described as 'Anime'.

Answer print. The first projection print of an edited film from a film laboratory which includes a synchronized sound track and colour corrected scenes.

Antagonist. The person element or force which opposes the central character of a film in his efforts to achieve a goal.

Anticlimax. (In film script). Ineffective end to anything that has suggested a climax.

Aperture. (F-#, F-stop, Effect aperture, Relative aperture).— Effective size of the lens opening through which light passes on the film. The ratio of focal length of a lens to its effective aperture for an object located at infinity is called f/number or relative aperture. The apparent diameter of a lens viewed from the position of the object against a diffusely illuminated background is called the effect aperture.

Apple box. A multipurpose, hollow wooden cube used in film-production as stops, wedges, platforms etc.

Arranger. A musician who writes the harmonies and instrumental parts for the voicing of a musical piece. In Indian Hindi film music the names of Shamrao Kambale, Anil Mohile are recognised as stalwarts. Even celebrated Indian film director Satyajit Ray who has provided music to few of his Bengali films was also an arranger in his own way.

Art department. This department is principally responsible for the visual artistry required for the film on the floor. Ordinarily, Art department consists of the personel like art/assistant art/set directors, production buyer/designer, special effect supervisor, draftsman, set dresser, property master, leadman, swing gang and property assistant.

Art director. The person who oversees the film-artists and crafts people who build the sets for the film. In most of the European countries the Art director is known as 'Architect' or 'Decorateur'.

Artifact. (Artefect). A visual defect in an image caused by the limitations or the malfunction of imaging equipment. Product of human art and workmanship.

Artificial light. Light that emanates from any source other than the sun or sky.

ASCAP. The American Society of Composers, Authors & Publishers.

Aspect ratio. (Aspect/Academy Ratio). A measure of the relative sizes of the horizontal and vertical components of an image. Thomas Edison established silent film's academy ratio at 1.33:1. Anamorphic (35 mm) was set at 2.35:1.

ASA rating. (Also ANSI rating). A numerical rating of the sensitivity of film emulsion to Light as determined by erstwhile American Standards Association (ASA).

Assembly. The first stage in cutting after synchronizing the rushes.

Assistant Cameraman. (Asst. Camera Operator, First Asst., Cameraman, Asst. Camera, Camera Asst.). A member of the camera crew who assists the camera operator. Ordinarily, Asst. cameraman is responsible for the maintenance and care of the camera, as well as preparing dope sheets. In smaller camera screws, Assistant cameraman has also to perform the duties of clapper-loader and/or focus puller.

Assistant Director (AD). (First Asst. Director). An assistant director's duties include tracking the progress of filming. Also organising any large crowd scenes. He gives the commands to start filming and sound recording for the takes of the films.

Assistant film editor. (Assistant Picture/Sound/First/Second Asst./Apprentice Editor). He is responsible for providing any and all required logistical assistance to the editor/s. A member of the unit responsible for the smooth performance of the film's team.

Assistant Production Manager (Asst. Production Co-ordinator). An assistant to the production co-ordinator.

Associated Producer. A producer who shares responsibility for the film's creative and business issues.

Associated British Picture Corporation (ABPC). The production Division of the Associated British Corporation (1926).

Association Internationale du film d'Animation. (ASIFA). International Animation Association. ASIFA was founded in France in 1960. Chartered under UNESCO, as a membership organisation devoted to the encouragement and dissemination of film animation as an art and communication form.

Association of Film Commissioners' International (AFCI). A non-profit educational organisation founded in 1975 to serve the needs of on-location film, television and commercial film production.

Association of Film, Television & Radio Artists (AFTRA). An association with jurisdiction over some works that can be recorded by picture or by sound. The working of AFTRA is also equal to the working of Screen Actors Guild (SAG).

Association of Motion Picture & Television Producers (AMPTP). An Association created to facilitate motion picture and television producers for promoting activities at national and international levels.

Asynchronous sound. All sound which is relevant to the circumstances of a shot but which is not synchronised to the action.

Atmosphere. The mood or ambiance of a scene created in a production. Term also refers to extras that are selected for filming in a scene.

Audio. Sound, including dialogue, voice-over narration, music and effects.

Australian Screen Editors. (ASE). A cultural, professional and educational organisation, dedicated to the pursuit and recognition of excellence in the arts, sciences and technology of motion picture film and television post production. ASE's role is significant in promoting, improving and protecting in relations to screen productions.

Australian Society of Cinematographers. (ACS). This society was founded in Australia to bring together all the Australian cinematographers working in all branches of the film industry. Use of the abbreviation i.e. ACS after a name of the member of the society in the credit title of the film or for that matter in any document written/produced by ACS member indicates that the person is the recognised member of the ACS.

Automatic Dialogue Replacement. (ADR). (Dialogue Looping, Looping). The re-recording of dialogue by actors of a film or/and participants in the documentary films in a sound during post-production. Ordinarily ADR is perform to play-back of duly edited picture in order to match lip movements on screen. ADR enables to change the delivery or infection of a line. At times new lines of dialogue are conceived during the stages of editing. Due to the advantage of ADR these lines are in a position to incorporate by not showing the face of the actor concerned on the screen. The purpose of ADR is to replace the production track of pure quality.

Automatic Dialogue Replacement Editing. (ADR Editing). The process of editing sound of the film during ADR.

Automatic Dialogue Replacement Editor. (ADR Editor). The person who performs ADR editing under the patternal guidance of the chief film editor.

Automatic Dialogue Replacement Mixer. (ADR Mixer). The person who mixes the sound during ADR session.

Available Light. This term refers to the light existing naturally within a given area.

Avant-Garde. Term used loosely to describe any experimental movements in the arts, working outside or a opposition to accepted forms dealing with odd unsuitable subjects.

AVID. Manufacturer of a popular non-linear editing system. The term AVID is very often referred to the system itself as 'AVID editor.'

B

B. A letter in edit decision list (EDL) indicating that the edit is both an audio and video edit.

b.g. A script abbreviation for background.

Babble. Active voices with no discernable words are referred to as (crowd) babble.

Baby spot. Small type of spotlight for highlighting.

Back Projection. (Rear Projection). This term refers to the photographic technique which enables the photographer to film live action in front of screen which the background action is projected on. Originally this technique was used for scenes occurring in running vehicles.

Background Artist (Backgrounds, Scenic Artist). An artist responsible for designing or constructing the matter/ art placed at the rear of a set.

Back light. A light thrown on foreground actors or objects from farther back in the set. Back light separates them from the background and gives an impression of depth to the picture.

Back-potch. The portion of the blanking interval from the end of the colour burst to the beginning of the picture signal.

Backlot. (Backlot). A large undeveloped area on studio property used for constructing large open-air sets; Also used for filming wilderness scenes.

Background. Actions, objects or setting farther from the camera in the given shot/s.

Baffles. Sound-absorbing panels designed to help control and keep sounds isolated in recording studios..

Ballet films. Ensemble of theatrical performance of dancing and mime to music and films. Pavlova's dancing in 'Immortal Swan' (1936 is considered as early effort in Ballet Films.

Balop. Balophion projector, used in live T.V. commercials which throws images on screen by reflectors.

Banned. In most of the countries there are either government or official movie classification boards who are responsible for determining the suitability of a movie for release in their respective country or region. Considering the after effects on the minds of the public also taking care of the prescribed norms these boards giving reasons occasionally block the release of a movie either in the cinema hall or on video. Very often, a banned movie will find its way around a ban by means of bootleg distribution.

Barney. A flexible water-proof covering for a motion picture cameras.

Bars and tone. A video and audio reference used to assure that chroma (colour), luminance and audio (sound) are kept consistent between pieces of production equipment and recorded segment of tapes.

Beam. The pick-up angle of the microphone within which that instrument functions at it greater efficiency.

Beat. A momentary pause in an actor's action or delivery of speech.

Behind the Scenes. The off-camera goings on associated with film-making. A documentary worth mentioning in this context is 'Hearts of Darkness: A Film-maker's Apocalypse in 1991.

Below the line costs. In films, other than Above-the line costs, all other expenses for editing, film, hotels, laboratory, sound, technicians etc.

Best Boy (Girl). (Assistant Chief Lighting. Technician, Best Boy Grip, Best Boy Electric). The chief assistant, usually of the gaffer, but more often lately used as a general term for the second in command of a group. This term is likely borrowed from early sailing or whaling crews, as sailors were often employed to set up and work rigging in theatres. There are no 'best girls' per se; Female chief assistants are also called 'Best Boys'.

Betamix. Video cassette player developed and launched by SONY.

Bianco E Naro. Celebrated Italian monthly publication devoted exclusively to Films (1937-1951).

Bicycle Print. The (mal) practice of showing the same print (film) at more than one places on the same evening. In this process the bicycle-boys were employed on the mission of transporting the reels already shown to the next cinema houses for film exhibitions.

Big Close-up. (BCU). A shot of less that the complete head of the subject or a detail of an object. (Also known as 'extreme close up').

Billing. (Top/Diagonal/Equal Billing). A great deal of importance is placed on relative sizes, positions and order of names and movie's title in printed publicity material as well as the opening credits. Generally, higher positions designate higher importance. Additionally, there is significant given to the names which appear before or above the actual title of the movie. The person whose name is shown first in the credits or whose name is at the top of an advertisement is said to have received 'top billing'. Equal billing is recognised from the arrangement of giving the names of more than one artists. Here the importance of the people concerned decreases from left to right. In some movies with a large number of stars, the publicity department goes even to great lengths to satisfy the demands of various parties. 'Diagonal billing' is where a different names appears first, depending on whether the material is read from top to bottom, or from left to right. In some extreme cases, multiple stars in the same movie have each demanded to billing, in which case an equal number of differently-billed advertisement have been created.

Biograph. (In films) a camera and projector both in one.

Biographic picture. (Biopic) A filmed story of a person's life story.

Bioscope. The weekly trade journal of the cinema industry which was being published from London during 1908-1932, Mr. D.G. Phalke—father of the Indian films—was a regular reader of Bioscope, and he has had acknowledged his courtesy to the Bioscope in his articles and interviews.

Bipack colour. A process of natural colour cinematography.

Bipost Lamp. A globe having two pins on its base.

Bit part. A small unimportant role, usual lasting one scene.

Bits of Business. Actions or activities of actors within the scene. These may or may not be related to the principle action.

Black and White. (BW, B/W, B&W). In films this indicates that the images have no colour. As colour film stock had not been invented in early days the first movies were exclusively in black and white. Even after the invention of colour films and their uninterrupted availability some producers because of the artistic reasons of cheapness of price are still bringing out black and white films. Some films are shot using colour film stock but with the final print in black and white.

Black Comedy. A comedy in which the humour is derived from subjects which are typically considered 'serious', or for which humour is generally considered as unsuitable. Common examples of black comedy are death, war, suffering and murder.

Blacklisting. (Blacklist). A list of filmmakers or actors who have either been formally or informally discriminated against, due to their personal, political, social or religious beliefs. In 1950s in America, McCarthyism resulted in numerous filmmakers being blacklisted.

Blasting. To suddenly put more volume into the microphone or other transporting equipment than it can take Distortion invariably results.

Bleached out. A term used to describe a film or video image that has been overexposed and lacks overall density and detail.

Blimp. Sound absorbent box or cover fitted over a camera. It prevents the sound of the mechanism being picked up by the microphone while recording sound, with the picture.

Blockbuster. A movie which gains a huge financial success. In common usage a 'blockbuster' is a movie that has a box office of more than one hundred million dollars upon release in North America. A term 'blockbuster' came into increasing use in early sixties.

Blocking out the action. A film directors determination relating to the movement of the actors on the set.

Bloop. Opaque area over splice in positive sound track. This eliminates the click that which otherwise be produced.

Bloopin ink. Quick drying black opaque ink.

Blow-up. Converting 16 mm to 35 mm by laboratory process. In this process frame is optically enlarged so that the image is made to correspond to a closer shot.

Body Double. For some shots, a director of the film may consider that a particular actor's body may not be suitable for the impression desired. In these situations, the actor is 'doubled' (replaced) by a person whose body is more suitable. Typically, body doubles are used for shots requiring nudity or depictions of physical fitness. Body double is in contrast with stunt double and stand-in.

Body Make-up. Makeup applied below the neck or above the wrists.

Bollywood. A name ascribed to Indian film-world. Since Indian cinema is influenced by 'Hollywood' in many ways, it is being recognised as 'Bollywood' in recent times. The word 'Bolly' represents Bombay i.e. Mumbai, in general. In his author's note on the book entitled 'Follywood Flashback' Mr. Bunny Reuben writes that "Why Follywood Flashback?" Why not Bollywood Flashback, seeing as the name Bollywood has became widespread nomenclature for the Indian movie industry in recent times? No. It's not for merely for alliterative value. I was the originator of this nomenclature as Follywood for the Indian movie-industry as far back as forty years ago, when in 1952 I started a featurette....Most important, I think Bollywood is meaningless whereas, in one single word, Follywood subscribes it all."

Bomb. Bomb is a typical term is filmdom which has absolutely opposite meaning. In the United Kingdom 'bomb' means a rousing success while outside of the United Kingdom 'bomb' means a movie which is a financial disaster.

Boom Microphone. (Boom Mike, Boom). A long pole with a microphone on the end. The boom is extended out near the actors. Ideally, the microphone at the end should be placed in the camera's safe area.

Boom Operator. In film sound recording, a number of the sound crew who operates the boom microphone.

Booster light. Electrical lamps used to intensify daylight and to eliminate shadows.

Bootleg (smuggled) An unofficial and illegally copied or distributed version of a movie, very often of a substandard quality. Bootleg videos are often available for movies that have yet to be released in a particular country, or have been banned.

Box Office. (B.o., BO, Gross) A measure of total amount of money paid by cinema-goers to view a movie.

'B' Picture. A feature film made at a low cost and the limited length running into 55 to 75 minutes.

Breakdown. (Breakdown script). A detailed list of all items, people, properties, equipment etc. required for a scheduled shoot on a day-by-day basis. Recording such lists and keeping the same ready at the time of shooting proves to be useful and handy in maintaining the continuity and allows optimization of the time of the actors and the entire crew.

Breakdown Notes. In film music, the minute timing in seconds and tenth of seconds of a scene to be underscored.

Bridging shot. The kind of shot that allows a smoother or more acceptable transition than a direct cut.

British Board of Film Censors. (BBFC). This Board was set up in 1912 to approve films for public viewing. The Board works independently of the industry and of Government.

British Film Commission. (BFC). The British Film Commission is a Government funded organisation established in 1991, as an initial point of contact to assist in the making of international and domestic film and television throughout every step of production in England, Northern Ireland, Scotland and Wales.

British Film Institute. (BFI) was founded in 1933. It exists to promote greater understanding and appreciation of, and access to, film and moving image culture in the UK. An exclusive account of BFI's history has been brought out by Ivan Butler way back in 1971.

Broadway Melody. Metro-Goldwyn-Mayer (MGM) in 1928, when sound was first introduced for the first time in films, began with the 'Broadway Melody'. Eventually a cycle of such back-stage musicals was produced by MGM 'Broadway Melody', 'You were meant for Me', 'Singing in the Rain' are some of the world-known titles in the series.

Build-up. In film editing, cutting leading to a climax in the action.

Business. Action introduced in order to build-up or reinforce characterization, a sequence, a plot point or the like.

Butt Splice. A joint between two pieces of film without an overlap facilitated by the application of tape across the end frame of each section.

Butterfly. A large net or silk stretched of a frame and supported by a single stand commonly used outdoors to shade or diffuse direct sunlight.

Butterfly Lighting. A type of portrait lighting popularized by George Hurrell and other glamour in the year 1930.

"Buy". A director's term of acceptance for a shot. (Also called 'circled Take').

Buzz Track. Sound that represents the 'presence' in a room or space in which a recording usually of a voice/s has been made. It is used for spacing or extending pauses when track laying and is a non-synchronized track.

C

Cable. The connecting links between lamps and electrical sources, between television cameras and recorder or transmitting between the mikes and the sound recorder.

Caldwell Halo Screen. This screen operates on the principle of rear and side lighting and has the projection screen hanging in the mid air. All supports for this screen are invisible to the audience.

Calibrations. The marks on lens barrels denoting the size of iris stop being used for photography.

Call sheet. A listing of which actors will be required for which scenes, and when they will be required on set/ location scheduled for film-shooting. Call sheets are created by assistant directors and other responsible persons connected with the film-shooting. Ordinarily, these call-sheets indicate the work to be performed on the next day.

Cameo. A bit part played by a famous actor who would ordinarily not accept such a small part. Originally meaning 'a small piece of art work. The term 'cameo' was borrowed by film director Michael Anderson when he was attempting to attract famous actors to play bit parts in his famous film 'Around the World in 80 Days' (1956). In this film cameos from an all-star cast supported David Niven, Cantinflas, Shirley MacLaine and Robert Newton. (term 'cameo' is derived from a small piece of relief-carving in stone, usually with colour layers utilized to give background relief design of smaller form.)

Camera. A device/apparatus for taking images/photographs.

Camera Crew. The group of crew members directly involved with operation of the camera. Individual job titles include: clapper-loader, camera operator, assistant cameramen, director of photography, focus puller, grip, key grip, dolly grip, additional camera.

Camera Identification Marks. To enable to know at a glance in what camera the film has been shot through these marks of special design are cut into the side of the camera aperture gate of standard 8 mm and 16 mm cameras.

Camera Loader. (Clapper-Loader, Clapper Loader). The person who operates the clapboard at the beginning of a shot. Camera Loader is also responsible for loading film stock into film magazines. The action of slapping the clapper was invented as a way of synchronizing the visual and audio components of a shot. Recent innovations in audio-visual synchronization have made this sort of action unnecessary, but even today it still occurs extensively.

Camera Obscura. Darkened box with aperture for projecting image of distant object on screen within.

Camera Operator. (Cameraman). The person of the film unit who operates the camera while shooting. He/she has to operate the camera to the prescribed specifications dictated by the director of photography. A director or a director of photography sometimes assumes this role. It is a shown fact that director Luc Besson always operates the camera on films he directs.

Camera Rehearsal. A staging of the action of the shot or scene with actors or stand-ins that also includes camera movements.

Camera Report. A report of negatives which includes all pertinent information required for laboratory and editing department of the film.

Camera shots. These are ordinarily divided into four groups viz. angle shot, pan shot, tilting shot and tracking shot.

Camp. (Campy). A form of comedic parody where the cliched conventions of a dramatic form like adventure are deliberately exaggerated to the point of ridiculousness.

Canadian Film Development Corporation. (CFDC). This was set up in early 1967 with a fond of $ 10 million to promote the feature film industry of Canada.

Canadian Society of Cinematographers. (CSC). Use of the abbreviation after a name indicates that the person is a member of the CSC.

Caper Film. An adventure film generally presented from thieves' part of view.

Caption. Title, descriptive text or translation placed between shots or superimposed on them.

Carbon Arc. Most frequently used for film and television work (225 amp Brute).

Carry on. British-made series of formula comedy films. In 1958 Peter Rogers produced his first such film in the series entitled 'Carry on Sergent'. By the end of 1974 he produced 26 such films in the series for which Gerald Thomas exclusively shared the responsibility of direction for all these films.

Cartage. (In music). The pick-up and delivery of musical instruments to and from recording sessions.

Cast. A collective term for the actors (characters) appearing in a particular movie.

Cast List. A list frequently giving brief description of the roles in a film.

Casting. The process of hiring actors to play the characters in a script, typically done by a casting director, but with some input from a director, producer, or studio.

Casting Agent. The person who arranges for casting interviews and conducts negotiations with the actor's/ representative in accordance with guide lines set by the Producer.

Casting Couch. During the so-called "Golden Age" of Hollywood, it was not very uncommon for would-be-stars to grant sexual favours to director and/or producers of a film in return for a role in films. These favours were usually rumoured to be on a couch in the film-makers' office. Since then the phrase 'casting couch' has been popularized, and although that old practice has diminished, the term still remains in use in filmdom.

Casting Director. (Casting Assistant, Casting Associates, Extras Casting). While planning for the film, directors and producers rely heavily on the Casting Director to assist them with assembling the perfect cast for their production. Casting Director auditions and helps to select all of the speaking role actors in film, television shows or theatrical plays. The Casting Director is always expected to possess a vast knowledge of the actor pool He has to be able to match a variety of actors with just the right type of role. Casting Directors are also responsible for providing their services as the liaison between the director and the actors and their agents. Casting directors negotiate the deals with the agents of the actors as soon as the actors have been cast in the film under production and are also responsible for the contracts.

Casting Society of America. (CSA). With the intention of working efficiently and smoothly Casting Directors working in theatre, film and television have formed this Society. Since CSA is not an official union or a guild, every Casting Director working in these mediums is not necessarily a member of organisation. Even then American film directors/producers give preference to CSA members, as and when it is possible.

Catalytic Event is that critical event that precipitates the main character's action. In short film the catalytic event is central, as it precipatates the story.

Caterer (Catering). A person or company who provides the main meals for cast and crew either on set or on location. This is considered to be a highly professional job. For the purpose of snack service 'craft service' is also provided by the same or other caterers.

Cathod ray tube. A special type of vacuum tube wherein electrons emitted from a cathode are concentrated into a beam and caused to play upon a special screen which glows at the point of impact.

Cel. (Cell). A hand-drawn sheet representing a single animation frame usually made of a clear material like cellulose or mylar, to allow several layers of composition. Cell animation allows an artist to draw the stationary elements once for each scene and in this process only moving images are drawn 60 times on 60 cells.

Cell-side. The opposite side to the emulsion on a piece of film, usually recognizable because it is shiny and reflective.

Censorship. (Censoring Censor). Changes required of a movie by some person or body other than the studio or the filmmakers, usually a national or regional film classification board. (See also Certificate). In India, the system of provincial censorship of films has been in force since the days of the Indian Cinematographic Act in 1918.

Central Censor Board. (Indian). The Board established in 1951 with its headquarters in Mumbai (than Bombay), the regional offices at Calcutta and Chennai (then Madras). This system classify films into 2 groups and issues Universal/Adult Certificates for the purpose of releasing films.

Centre International du Film pour l'Enfance et al. Jeunesse. (C.I.F.E.J./CIFEJ International Centre of Films for Children and Young People). This international non-Government organization whose goal is to promote only quality films, television programmes and videos for children and young people around the world.

Certificate/s. (Rating/s). Various countries or regions have film classification boards for reviewing movies and rating their content in terms of its suitability for particular audiences. For many countries, movies are required to be advertised and announced as having a particular 'certificate' or 'rating', for warning audiences of possible 'objectionable content' (See also Censorship).

Certificate of Origin. This states in the body of the certificate country's origin of a picture and is usually a notarized statement.

Chalk marks. These marks on the flow indicate the actors as to where they should end movement made on the set.

Channel. A sub-division on a reel of magnetic tape.

Change Pages. When a script is being edited during the production of a film various changes are distributed to actors and the filmmakers on 'change pages' which are usually a different colour to the pages of the script.

Change-Over Marks. (Change-Over, Reel Change, Reel Change Marks). Most completed movies consist of more than one reel, and thus for an un-interrupted Screening, at least two projectors must be used. Towards the end of a reel, one or more frames may include a small circle in one of the corners. These are signals to the projectionists that the current reel is approaching the end and she/he should be ready to start the next projector, which should have the next reel prepared for projection.

Change Room. Fully equipped editing room where film editor can make last minute changes.

Changing bag. A slight-proof bag used for loading or unloading magazines with films.

Character. A person in the film.

Character Actor. An actor who specializes in playing a particular style of a character. He is very often stereotypical, offbeat or humorous.

Characterization. Individual's details given by the script-writer.

Charlie Chan. The name of the Chinese detective drawn from Earl Derr Biggers popular novels. For the first consecutive 17 films actor Warner Oland played in this title role.

Cheat. The repositioning of a character or a subject in a way convenient for taking a shot that is not consisting with the positioning in other shots.

Checkboard Assembly. A system of assembling the masters of a film to enable dissolves to insert. In checkboard assembly joints are not seen in the print.

Childrens' Entertainment Films Division. (CEFD). Films Division exclusively for childrens' entertainment set up by Rank Organization in 1944. Mary Field was appointed as Director of this Division.

Childrens' Film Foundation. (CFF). This Foundation was established in United Kingdom for imparting training to school children. The main object of establishing the Foundation to provide experience of all aspects of film making along with developing film appreciation in children. The Foundation has been now replaced by the Children's Film and Television Foundation with a view to give accent on all aspects of television also.

Children's Film's length. Various countries have prescribed their **children's film length.** Govt. of India has decided that the length of the children's film should not be more than 8000 ft. This rule is not applicable for the feature films made in India wherein the children are playing the main rolls or/and full-length films based on juvenile literature.

Children's Film Society. (CFS). This Society was set up in 1955 in India. By the end of 1962 under the able guidance and directorship of Ezra Mir and also with the help of celebrated film directors from the film industry, Childrens' Film Society produced 16 featurette films and 12 short subjects. Thereafter new set up took place to accelerate this Society's activities.

Choreographer. A person who plans and directs dance sequence within a movie and supervises dances/mass movements.

Chute Cowboys. In films popular slang term for experienced parachutists that either perform or assist with stunts involving parachutes.

Child Stars. Considering the mass-appeal, Hollywood producers started taking child actors in this films, which proved to be very successful. This formula of engaging child stars for films became prevalent in the films world-over.

Cinch Marks. (Scratches). Scratches on a print running parallel to the edge of the strip of film. Typically caused by improper reel winding which allows one coil of the print to slide against another.

Cine Check. A device that reads and displays the frame rate of a video monitor used for synchronizing a motion picture camera with a video image.

Cinema. (1) A place where screenings occur. Cinemas can be hardtrops or ozoners. (2) Central Hall, Lancashire (Britain) is considered as the first Cinema House (1907)

(3) Italian Monthly Film Journal which was effectively being run during the period between 1936 and 1956.

Cinema Audio Society. (CAS). A philanthropic non-profit organization (NGO) formed in 1964 for the purpose of sharing information with Sound division professionals in the motion picture, television and now video industry. Use of the abbreviation after a name indicates that the person is a member of the CAS.

Cinema India. The monthly film magazine brought out by National Film Development Corporation, Nehru Centre, Mumbai. It offers a blend of articles, interviews and insights into filmcraft.

Cinema Verite. Literally cinema Truth. A documentary style in which no directorial control is exerted. The term is frequently misused to describe new-wave 'handheld' camera techniques. This style of film-making begun in Europe in 1950s.

Cinemascope. Novel photographic and sound system introduced by 20th Century Fox. Professor Henry Chretion —French expert — invented this system, and later Company technicians of 20th Century Fox studio perfected it. The first picture in cinemascope was 'The Robe' which presented on the screen two and half times large picture than ordinary size. This 1953 film made in the cinemascope process was based on the Bible story in which Richard Burton appeared as Gallio, a Roman tribune put in charge of the execution of Jesus Christ. The duration of this first film in cinemascope was of 135 minutes.

Cinematic Grammar. This is comprised action within the shots, angles, camera movements, music, shots etc.

Cinematographer. (Cinematography, Cin). A person with expertise in the art of capturing images either electronically or on film stock through the application of visual recording devices and the selection and arrangement of lighting. The chief cinematographer for a movie is called the Director of photography, and he is ultimately responsible for the process of recording a scene in the manner desired by the director of the film.

Cinema. In this system, picture presentation is accomplished through use of huge curved screen which provides a full vision of 146 degrees horizontally and 55 degrees vertically. Introduced for the first time on 30th September, 1952.

Cine-Roman. Novelettist films including serials. (French term coined around 1904).

Clap Board. (Clapper, Slate). A small board which holds information identifying a shot. It typically contains the working title of the movie, the names of the director and director of photography, the scene and take numbers, the date and the time. It is filmed at the beginning of a take. On the top of the clap board is a hinged stick which is often 'clapped' to provide audio/ visual synchronization. The basic aim of the clap board is to bring in synchronization process in the cutting room.

Clapper Boy. Junior technician who operates the clap board.

Classical Metronome. This mechanical box with tempos from 40 beats to 208 beats per minute is used by musicians to maintain tempo of the music.

Classification and Ratings Administration. (CARA). Motion Picture Association of America (MPAA) has established CARA as its division. CARA is basically responsible for administering the certificates to be issued by MPAA. In the latter part of 1968, MPAA introduced a rating system to enable people to judge what kind of audience a movie was meant for and whether or not it was okay to take the kids to see it along with them. The classification system now consists of five categories. "G" means general audience, people of any age may be admitted to see the film; "PG" indicates "Parental Guidance"; some material may not be suitable for children; "PG-13" is a new rating that strongly suggests parents give special guidance to children under 13; "R" indicates "Restricted", a person under 17 requires accompanying parent or adult guardian. "X" indicates no one under 17 admitted (age limit may vary in certain areas). CARA plays a pivotal role in identifying MPAA ratings. Sometimes some films are unrated. For example, 1984 film Bolero which was made as a vehicle to display Bo Derek's physical charms (It's highlight was Bo's brief sex scenes with a sheik and a bullfighter) contains nudity and simulated sex, is unrated. At times after due consideration some of the films are re-rated. For example, John Travolta-starrer 'Saturday Night Fever' (1977) directed by John Badham which was originally rated "R" was later released in a "PG" version to capture a younger audience. Some of the film-producing countries have started rating their national films on the guidelines of CARA.

Claymation. Animation of models constructed from clay or plasticine.

Clean Speech. A take in which all the dialogues are performed without a single error.

Click Track. A substitute for a metronome in the form of a sound track with regular clicks inserted, enabling the conductor to retain the correct tempo in recording music to the cut film.

Cliffhanger. A moment of gigh drama, frequently used at the end of serials. Named for the (now cliched) practice of leaving a hero or heroin onto the edge of a cliff.

Climax. The crises in the story, the high point in dramatic tension.

Clipping. A defect that occurs in video images that are overexposed.

Close Captioned. (CC). A system which displays the current dialogue on screen for deaf or hard-of-hearing viewers. (Not to mix with subtitles).

Close Shot. (CS). The term indicates that the camera is close to the subject.

Close Up. (CU). A shot in which the subject is larger than the frame, revealing much detain. The abbreviation is often used in a slug line.

Colonial Film Unit. (CFU). This was founded by William Seelors in 1939 as a part of Britain's Wartime Information Services (WIS).

Co-Producer. A film producer who has an equal responsibility for the completion of a project as per scheduled programme.

Code Numbers. (Also Edge Numbers or Rubber Numbers). A method of numbering films and/or magnetic stock to provide a reference for logging purposes.

Colour Consultant. A technical advisor with expertise in film stock and film developing, who provides advice for cinematographers and colour timers.

Colour Compensating Filters. Filters used on the film camera to adjust the colour temperature of the light that is required.

Colour Correction. The process by which the film is adjusted for correct colour balance in the printing.

Colour Gels. Sheets of coloured plastic material which modifies the colour of light.

Colour Rendering Index. (CR Index). A measurement with natural daylight and incandscent lighting. Only sources that measure go or higher are considered suitable for photographic applications.

Colour Temperature. In film photography this is a measure which defines the colour of the light source. The colour temperature is a means of expressing the colour quality/ source of light.

Colour Timing (Colour Correction, Colour Timer, Colour Corrected). A process which adjusts the final print so that colours match from shot to shot, regardless of the film stock and camera which is used to shoot the particular scene. The name colour shot is ascribed since one aspect is adjusting the exposure time of each shot. Colour timing process is performed by a colour timer.

Colourization. (Colourized). This is a film alteration process where an operator digitally alters a black and white image to include colour. It is a controversial practice because many film-makers and viewers believe it fundamentally alters an artistic creation. Early attempts at colourization in the 1980s were relatively crude in this shading range. Examples of this kind of alteration are versions of "Casablanca" (1942) and "It's a Wonderful Life" (1946). A film entitled "Citizen Kane" (1941) is notable in that Orson Welles was able to legally prevent its alteration.

Commage Print. A print with picture and magnetic sound combined on the same piece of film. This term was coined by British Broadcasting Company.

Compilation film. A film edited from material gathered from a number of sources on the same subject.

Completion Bond. The Bond which ensures that the film is physically completed. It, however, does not give guarantee to the effect of the films' artistic or creative value.

Composer. A musician whose music appears in the movie's score. Most of the movies have at least some original music written for the score, usually after the relevant parts of the movie have been filmed. Musical compositions consisting of words written by poets/song writers are known as lyrics.

Composite Print. (Also called synchronized Print). A print with images and sound on the same strip of film. The sound component may be either a magnetic soundtrack or an optical soundtrack. The distance between a point on the soundtrack and the corresponding image is called an advance of a composite print.

Composite Track. Any track that incorporates more than one element is called the composite track.

Composition. In photography, the framing of a picture area to achieve a desired distribution and balancing of light, mass, shadow, colour and movement.

Conductor. (Musical Conductor, Orchestra Conductor). The leader of the orchestra who directs the orchestra's performance of the score, often the composer. He establishes tempo by making definitive motions with a baton.

Confederation Internationale des Cinemas d'art et Essai (CICAE). International Confederation devoted to the cause of films and film-theatres.

Conforming. (In editing film process). Process of cutting master or original negative to match the cutting copy or work print in preparation for printing.

Confrontation. A unit of conflict and the main structural component of plot.

Construction Co-ordinator (Construction Foreman, Construction Manager). Financial responsibilities include budgeting, tracking costs, generating reports, etc. Through drawings, a construction co-ordinator is directed artistically by the Production Designer and Art Director to produce their "vision" in three dimensions. Construction Co-ordinator of the film unit is also responsible for the physical integrity of the structures built by the construction department.

Contact Printing. In photography the reproduction method whereby light is directed through a developed negative on an unprocessed positive film stock, each being in contact with the other.

Continuity. (Continuity cover). The degree to which a movie is self-consistent. For example, a typical scene where an actor is wearing a hat when seen from one camera angle and not from another camera would necessarily lack continuity. An exclusive person is employed very often for this special purpose and the duty of this person is to observe the continuity part of the scene shot. This is very essential as reshooting embarrassing lapses in continuity can be prohibitively expensive and also time consuming. By the virtue of digital composite process some continuity errors are being corrected in modern times. Particular scenes from "Terminator 2". Judgement Day" (1991) trivia entry is one such pertinent example.

Continuity is the British film term for story-line.

Continuity Cutting. In film editing, smooth logical flow that preserves the illusion of the reality.

Continuity Report. (Continuity Script). A detailed list of the events that occurred during the filming of a scene. Typically recorded are production and crew identification, camera settings, environmental conditions, the status of each take, and exact details of the action that occurs. By recording all possible sources of variation, the report helps cut down continuity error between shots or even during re-shooting. A continuity report from "Star Wars" (1977) for example.

Contrast. The relative difference between the darkest and lightest elements in an image or scene of a film.

Core. (Bobbin). A plastic centre on which film is wound.

Costume. The clothes worn by actors when being filmed.

Costume Designer. (Assistant Costume Designer). A person who designs the costume for a movie.

Costume Supervisor. A person who supervises and takes every care of costume during the scheduled programme of shootings.

Costumer. (Wardrobe, Assistant Wardrobe, Wardrobe Assistant). A person responsible for handling the costumes worn by actors.

'Cot-death' film. A movie declared as 'failed' by the audience at the very first review of it in the cinema-hall. The reasons for the failure of the movie in such cases can not be assumed or ascribed. In medical science the death of a young baby from no apparent disease is called 'cot-death'.

Crab Shot. A shot that includes a lateral movement from the side of the scene.

Cracks. (In music), any played or sung note that is out of pitch.

Craft Service. During film shooting the craft service is held responsible for maintaining a table of snacks between meal periods. Sometimes, Craft Service has to feed the entire crew or extras scheduled for the film shooting. (See also Caterer).

Crane Shot. A shot made with the camera mounted on a crane which affords an overall point of view.

Creator. (Concept). The writer or other primary creative force behind a film, series, episodes or group of characters.

Credits. The titles on a film which 'credit' crew and cast involved in the production.

Crewmembers. (Crew). A collective term for anyone involved with the production of a movie who does not appear in the movie. This term is usually used to refer to the more subordinate members of a production team. The term 'crewmembers' is in contrast with filmmakers.

Crises. A peak in a screen-play's development, brought on by a major threat to the protagonist's chances of attaining his story goal.

Critical angle. In photography, the smallest angle of incident light reflected onto an interior surface at which total internal reflection takes place.

Cross cut. In film editing while alternating from one scene to another two or more subjects are presented in fragments through cross cutting.

Cross Light. (In film photography). A type of light that takes across the subject. Cross Light tends to be one of the most evocative types of lighting.

'Crude'story. The one-line film story which is written in its natural unprocessed state.

Cue. A designation given to the scene or area of picture to be covered musically.

Cut. Instantaneous change in either camera or placement, location or time. 'Cut' is called during filming to indicate that the current take is over. At times cut is also called if the director or other responsible person on the spot feels that the scene being filmed is not upto the mark or faulty for various reasons. A cut of a movie is also a complete edited version.

Cutaway. In continuity of the film, cutting a shot which does not include any part of the preceding shot.

Cutin. Any shot filmed for cutting into a master scene.

Cutting copy. The work print of a film exclusively used for the purpose of film-editing.

Cute performance. A daintily or quantity pleasing shot or performance given by actor/s on the set while filming.

Cyanine. Any group of dyes used as sensitisers in photography.

Cyanotype. Blue print.

Cyberpunk. A subgence of science fiction that typically has elements which include a futuristic tone, massive urban areas in decay and poverty, partial environmental collapse, extremely powerful business corporations, random street gang violence with the overall presence of extremely powerful computer, robotic and information technology. "Blade Runner" (1982) is considered the definitive cyberpunk movie.

Cycle. In film music a group of songs with related subjects.

Cyclops images. In documentary films prehistoric style of masonary with immense stones of irregular form.

Cyclorama. A circular panorama. A curved background in stage and cinematographic sets, used to give impression of sky distance and for lighting effects.

D

Dailies. (Rushes). The first positive prints made from the negatives photographed on the previous day. During filming sessions, the director, producer, distributc: or/ and some actors may view these dailies as an indication of how the filming and the actors' performances are progressing.

Day for Night. Daylight exterior shots simulating night by means of filters.

Decible. (dB) is one tenth (1/10) value of bel (10 decible). This numerical or dimensionless quality is a measure of power difference. Decibel is a unit for expressing the intensity of soundson a scale from zero for the average least perceptible sound to about one for the average pain level.

Decoupage. The design of a movie, the arrangement of shots.

Deferments. When an actor accepts a postponed payment of a part or entire salary.

Denoument. The concluding scenes of a movie where the story elements are finished and the characters' status after the climax is shown.

Demille's Dictum. Cecil B. Demille (1881-1959) the celebrated American film personality visited India in 1957. He became constant inspiration for Indian film Producers and Directors who maintained that every feature film should necessarily have a good story which could be acquired from any source like old epics, good authors or/and newspaper clippings. The prize-winning entry in a newspaper's film idea competition was instrumental in producing a picture like 'Ten Commandments' which proved to be very successful at box office wherever it was released.

Density. The variable degree of light-stopping power in a photographic image.

Depth of Field. (DoF). A measure of the length along a camera's line of site in which objects will be in focus. Distance from the nearest to the furthest points.

Depth of Focus. The range of focal planes behind the lens at the film plane. (Not to confuse with Depth of Field).

Detailed Budget. A complete cost analysis of the entire production of a picture.

Dialogue Coach. (Dialogue Director, Dialect Coach). A person who helps an actors speech for their character, Usually Dialogue Coach is found essential for assisting the actors in explaining the nuances of the language (spoken word) and showing accents and pronunciation.

Dialogue Editor. A sound editor assigned for the film who specializes in editing dialogue.

Dialogue Trainer. In certain film productions this post is filled by the producers to guide and train the actors on the sets while having conversations between the two or more persons. In certain units a Dialogist is specially appointed who is a speaker in, or writer of dialogues.

Dichroic Filter. In film photography, filter is used in front of lamps to adjust their colour temperature to that of daylight.

Dick-film. A slang used for detective film.

Diffusers. Gelatines or screens used to soften harsh lights.

Digital Audio Tape. (DAT). A small high-capacity tape that stores its data digitally.

Digital compositing. A technique whereby separately filmed components are combined through digital editing. (Not to confuse with optical printing).

Digital Computer. A computer that operates with numbers expressed as discrete pulses representing digits. An electronic precision calculating machine using arithmetical digits, generally binary or decimal notation.

Digital Editing. Editing a portion of a movie by digitizing one or more frames and altering them electronically or combining them with other digitized images. Thereafter the work of printing the modified frame is taken up.

Digital Metronome. An electronic box with metronomic settings based on frames of film and a frame's division into 8ths.

Digital Theatre Systems. (DTS). Companies like Dolby Digital, SDDS which have produced a digital soundtrack standards.

Digital Versatile Disc. (Digital Versatile Video Disc, DVD) Digital Versatile Discs (DVD) resemble audio CDs in appearance but have a much higher storage capacity. Therefore, these discs can store rich digital media such as video in addition to audio and computer software. DVD was previously called 'Digital Video Disk' but this new name changed reflects its wider uses. As a video medium, digital versatile disc offers full-length feature films to be stored with exceptional picture quality accompanied by high and digital sound, such as DTS and Dolby Digital. Because of its advantage of high capacity of discs, digital versatile discs movies are very often sold with extra features such as the option to view the movie in widescreen or full screen, or the option to listen to the movie or direct commentaries.

Dimmer. A bank of rheostans used to adjust intensity of light.

Dinky inky. A 150 or 200 watt bulb used to highlight certain scenes from the films.

Direct Cinema. A documentary style that has been dominant since the 1960s. The name was given by Albert Maysles. Direct cinema its viewers emphasis to the work without preconceived ideas. Besides less importance is given to the technical side.

Direct Cut. Cut to next numerical take.

Directing Animator. The animator who is responsible for creating the key poses or key frames of an animation.

Director. (Dir, Helmer) Director of the film is always a principal creative artist on a movie set. Not always, but usually the film's Director is the driving artistic source behind the filming process, and communicates to actors that way that he/she would like a particular scene played. A Director's duties might also include casting, script, editing, shot selection, shot composition and editing. Ordinarily, a Director has complete artistic control over all aspects of the movie in hand and under production. In some cases, in order to keep up busy schedule or the facilitate to shoot at two different places simultaneously a Direct assigns part of his job to his assistant for filming particular scenes in the film by forming a second unit.

Director of Photography. (DP, DoP). A cinematographer who is ultimately responsible for the process of recording a scene in the manner and style desired by the director of the film. Selection of film stock, cameras, lenses, designing and selecting lighting, directing the gaffer's placement of lighting shot composition, film developing and film printing are some of the many numbers of possible duties of the Director of Photography. Most of these duties are to be performed by him in consultation with the director of the film.

Director's Cut. (DC). Director's cut is fully edited and has a synchronized soundtract. This cut is usually not colour corrected or density corrected and may not even have the final music and effects tracks. In more recent times, the term Director's cut has taken on a popular meaning that implies a polished final cut of the movie that the director has complete artistic control over. Prevalent contracts under the terms of the Hollywood Director's Guild (HDG) usually allow six weeks for a director to assemble a cut of a movie without studio interference as she would like it to be seen.

Director's Guild of America. DGA An organization established by the professional American Film Directors.

Directorate of Film Festivals. (DFF). This Directorate was established by Ministry of Information and Broadcasting of Government of India. Its present address is Directorate of Film Festivals, Ministry of I & B., Govt. of India, Lok Nayak Bhavan, 4th Floor, Khan Market, New Delhi—110 003 (India).

Directors Guild-Producer-Training Plan. (Director's Guild of America Trainee, DGA Trainee) This Guild has various training programmes, and students can gain experience working in the film or television by working in various production divisions.

Dirty Dupe. An expensive black and white film useful for sound mixing or/and editing. It protects the edited work print.

Discontinuity. A fault in the continuity during the filming of a scene.

Disk. (Also Disc) A round flat plated coated with a magnetic substances on which data for a computer is stored.

Disc pack. A computer storage device consisting of a stack of discs, rotating at high speed, each disk having its own head to read and write data.

Dissolve. (Lap dissolve). An editing technique whereby the image of one shot is gradually replaced by the image of another. Commonly used for transition through time and or space between sequences.

Distribution Deal. A contract to distribute the film to exhibitors in specified territories.

Distribution Strategies, New. In order to reach the largest possible audience, Indian cinema has continued to expand; capitalizing on new distribution strategies. 'The Macmillan International Film Encyclopedia' mentions that the film 'Maine Pyar Kiya/I fell in love (directed by Sooraj Barjayta) remained the number one box-office draw for several years in the early 90s. It was simply re-cut and re-edited every few months, with new bits and pieces and then re-distributed to an adoring public.

Distributor. (Distrib, Distribution). An agent or the organization responsible for co-ordinating the distribution of the finished movie to exhibitors, as well as the sale of videos, laser-disks and other media versions of movies.

Documentary. (Docu). A non-fiction narrative film without actors. Typically a documentary is a journalistic record of an event, person, or place. In the beginning documentary was known as an actuality film. First documentary films were of shorter duration. Charles Urban's Kinemacolour presentation of 'Delhi Durbar' (1911) had a longer i.e. two and half hours duration. Considering the aspects of usefulness, informative value, impact of propaganda on the minds of the spectators, documentary films became popular world-over. In India, Documentary Film Festivals are becoming more and more popular and celebrated Directors also take pride in directing such documentaries under their able direction.

Dolby Noise Reduction. (Dolby, Dolby Labs, Dolby Digital, Dolby SR, Dolby 70 mm, Dolby). Dolby Laboratories, Inc. has produced a number of noise reduction and sound enhancement processes.

Dolby System. A proprietary noise reduction system, first developed for tape and cassette recording and now applied to 35 mm films.

Dolly. (Dolly shot, Dolly up, Dolly in, Dolly back, Pull back). A dolly is a small wheeled camera platform oriented truck which rolls along dolly tracks carrying the camera. The action of moving the camera towards or away from the object that it is pointing at is possible because of the mobility of 'Dolly'. The functions of Zoom and Dolly are quite different in as much as the fact that in a zoom, the relative positions and sizes of all objects in the frame remains the same, whereas in a dolly shot it changes as the camera moves. In his film entitle 'Vertigo' Alfred Hitchcock used a combination zoom—in and dolly back, resulting in a dramatic change in perspective.

Dolly Grip. A grip that moves a dolly.

Dolly Tracks. A set of tracks upon which a camera can be moved.

Donald Duck. One of the prominent character of Walt Disney's cartoon films. First appeared in 'The Wise Little Hen' (1934).

Dope Sheet. (Camera Report). A list of scenes from the script that have already been filmed, on a list of contents of an exposed reel of film stock. An accurate dope sheet is the responsibility of the Assistant Cameraman.

Doppler. Change in a quality of sound approaching and leaving as occurs when an airplane flies overhead.

Doppler Effect. A change in the apparent frequency of sound, light or other waves when there is relative motion between the source and the observer.

Double. A stand-by or replica (duplicate made by original artist of his picture etc.) In music, an orchestra member who plays more than one instrument.

Double Bill. Two movies shown consecutively, typically for a discounted single admission price. Very often these movies are sequels or are otherwise related with each other.

Double Head Projector. A film projector with facility for projecting separately and simultaneously positive image back and sound track.

Double System. A sound film system in which picture and sound are recorded on separate but precisely synchronized reels of film.

Down. A film term used for reducing volume of music or sound effects.

Down beat. The first beat of any beat of music.

Draftsman. While preparing the paper work of the scheduled film, a person who creates the planes for set construction.

Dream Mode. In this images are unconnected and very much lack the logical continuity; supposedly how mind works.

Drive in. A form of outdoor cinema in which patrons watch the film from their own cars. (Like drive-in hotels).

Driver. (A transportation Captain). A person who drives either equipment or passenger trucks, typically between location shootings, sets and the audio. The chief driver is called the Transportation Captain.

Drop-shadow. Used in titling to improve definition of lettering especially when titles are superimposed over live action backgrounds.

Dry run. Last rehearsal before shooting with empty camera with all lights, focus, action etc.

Dubbing. (Dubs, Dubbed). The technique of combining multiple sound components into one. The term is also used to refer to automatic dialogue replacement of a new language. In the United Kingdom the term 'dubbing' is commonly applied to the process of mixing of re-recording the various voices, effects, and also music tracks into a single master track, which occurs in all films. A layman finds dubbing as a useful means of translating foreign films into his own language. This is usually done after the film is completed, outside the country of origin and obviously without the supervision of the original director who has directed the film.

Dufay colour. A process of the thirties incorporation in the stock and a finally-ruled screen offered, blue and green lines. Humphrey Jenning's Design for Spring' (1938) is considered as fine Dufay colour film produced in thirties.

Dulling Spray. An aerosol spray that is applied to shiny items seen in a video picture, cuts down on glare and thus reduces hot spots.

Dummy. A machine that reproduces the sound one track.

Dunning Process. An early method of filming actors in the studio against a moving background photographed earlier.

Dupe. (Duping). To make or making of the duplicate material from an existing negative, print or reversal master.

Dupe Negative. This is taken from an original negative.

Dutch Tilt. A shot composed with the horizon not parallel with the bottom of the frame. United States' Director and actor Orson Welles (Citizen Kane-famed) has extensively and frequently used Dutch tilting method in films like 'Touch of Evil' (1958), 'Trail' (1963) etc.

Dye-transfer. A system of printing that involves the production of 3 colour separation positives. (Yello, cyan and magenta).

Dynamic frame. Edison's Kinetograph had a fixed shape in the horizontal 4:3 ratio derived from classical proportions dating back to the ancient Greeks.

Dyvour film company. The film company which has been declared as bankrupt.

E

Earwig. A small ratio receiver that fits into the ear.

Echo Chamber. A device used to give recording a hollow.

Edge Numbers. The numbers printed on the edge of a print. These allow easy identification of frames.

Edge Stripe. A magnetic stripe used to carry sound as an alternative to optical sound, usually in combined prints.

Edit Decision List. (EDL). The print out and/or disc that contains the edit information to recreate a video programme.

Editing. (Visual/Film Editing). Reconstructing the sequence of events in a movie. The very earliest, films were simple uncut shots strung together. Stalwarts like Edwin Porter, Cecil Hepworth and D.W. Griffith developed film narrative by cutting method. Before the introduction of sound, editing was generally used to strengthen the elements that were available in films. The technique of film-editing was furthered by implementing the process of assembling the individual shots and sound tracks made for a film into a coherent whole. A book entitled 'The technique of film editing' written by British Director Karel Reisz' (first published in 1953) is considered as 'Bible' on film editing.

Editing. Hints for. Creative contribution of the Editor of any film is good as the creative contribution of Director. Considering this aspect most of the world-known film-editors have given the following hints to the aspirants:

- Never allow a shot to remain unduly long on the screen,
- A shot or take that is not good or found useless should be stored under subject headings and not to be thrown away. Because these shots may also be useful in emergency cases,
- Always splice a good length of blank film on the beginning of a reel. The leader should be of five feet in length,
- There should be a good length of blank at the end of a reel, known as a trailer. It may not be as long as a leader but three feet will prove to be better,
- Never cut a tilting or panning shot unless tilting or panning is completed. But tilting or panning can be mixed with another tilting or panning shots, keeping the beginning frame and last frame steady,
- Always make a hard and fast rule of providing a white leader and a black trailer,
- To enable to indicate to the projectionist that the reel has been rewound, write the title of the film on the white portion of the leader,
- Provide a change over clue at the end of each reel by punching a hole usually in the top right hand corner of 4 or 5 frames just before the end of the last shot,
- Hanging over the shots must be very smooth to the eyes. That means that a long shot should be followed by midlong shot, then a mid shot and then a close shot. Close shot should never followed by a long shot, as long what should never be followed immediately by a close shot, so order of

joining the shots will roughly be as (i) long shot, (ii) medium shot, (iii) medium close shot (iv) close up (v) medium shot, and (vi) long shot, and so on,

- While joining two shots in which there is movement, it is necessary to place them side by side in order to find out two frames that will match. Cut would be made exactly there,
- The character should have the same expression and be in very nearly the same attitude at the point of joining, if shots are to match correctly,
- Find the best point at which to change from one camera angle or distance to another,
- Match the action from shot to shot,
- Judge the time a shot should remain on the screen,
- A simple subject should remain on the screen for only a short time and the subject containing much detail should remain longer,
- Shots in which the subject moves out of the frame should be cut just before the screen becomes empty,
- When splicing sound film it is better to paint the sound track with blooping ink or with black film to reduce the noise during projection,
- When cutting an action the movement of the character should be slightly more advanced at the beginning of the second shot than at the end of the first,
- To give emphasis to a particular situation the action should be broken up into series of shots,
- When cutting an action the movement of the character should be slightly more advanced at the beginning of the second shot than at the end of the first,

- Avoid using the same device too often,
- One shot should not be followed by 180 degree angle shot,
- Do not follow a left hand pan with a right hand pan unless there is special reason for doing so.

Editor. A person who performs editing in consultation with the director on a movie. This term usually refers to someone who does visual editing.

Effects. Recorded noises other than music or speech.

Effect Track. Sound track containing sounds other than music or speech.

8 mm. This smallest standard film of normally of 8 millimetres which was very first introduced in 1932 as an amateur film. Because of its easy handling, 8 mm films, became very popular amongst educational film agencies. In 1965, 8 mm was itself replaced by Super-8 and is now very much obsolescent. 8mm film was for some time being copiously used for rented cartoons.

Eire mob. The mobile or fickle common people are very often required by the film-makers to participate as 'Extra' in the films. Numerous American and British film-producers have safely depended on the Eirish mob for this purpose. Due to the comparatively cheap labour and also the spectacular scenery these producers have given their performance to the Fire mob.

Emulsion. Sensitive light substance which is coated on the film on one side. This carries the image or picture in a processed film. The top layer of the film.

Epic. To select a good story for the film is always one of the major tasks before the film-producers. In such cases classic epics come very handy. Since these are having large dramatic scope.

Episode Film. A collection of short fiction films by or more directors. These are usually grouped by a common author/theme to form a feature-length film.

Episodic. Script or film structure giving strong emphasis to incidence.

Equalization. The use of various electronic filters at the time of recording or mix to reduce unwanted frequences of noise.

Equity. (Actors equity). A trade union for actors. In the United Kingdom an organization entitled 'British Actors Equity Association (BAEA) has been established. According to the rules of BAEA any British actor is supposed to belong to Equity before being allowed to perform in any 'legitimate' theatre or film. Similar organisations exist in other countries but because other organisations often exist, membership is not as essential.

Establish. To make clear any element important to understanding and appreciation of a sequence or film.

Establishing Shot is used to establish a new scene.

Executive Producer. (Executive in charge of production) A producer who is not involved in any technical aspects of the filmmaking process. However, he is still responsible for the overall production. Ordinarily, an executive producer handles business and legal issues pertaining to the film-production.

Exhibitor. In films a person or/and organisation representing cinema.

Exploitation film. A low-budget movie produced for a specialized audience like horror fans etc.

Export of Indian Films. These are canalized through Indian Motion Pictures Export Corporation (IMPEC) which is a quasi-Government body. This is to streamline exports, avoid underhand dealings and promote cultural relationship. By the end of December 2000 Indian films were exported to over 100 countries. Keeping in view the popularity of Indian feature films in various countries, the National Film Development Corporation (NFDC) has been advised by Indian Parliamentary

Standing Committee to step us in exports of Indian films. Measures which could help raise the 0.1 per cent share of Indian cinema in the international market include market survey for exploring the possibilities to export Indian films, overseas acquisition of video rights and satellite broadcast/telecast rights.

Exposition. The early scenes in a film which lay the foundations of situation and characters in the plot.

Exposure. The amount of light which is allowed to reach a single frame of film while shooting.

Exterior. (EXT). Used in a slug line, indicates that the scene occurs outdoors. In other words, film shots/scenes made out-of-doors.

Extra. A person who necessarily appears in a movie where a non-specific, non-speaking character is required, usually as part of a crowd or in the background of scene. Extras are often recruited from wherever they are available. Please refer to EIREMOB. Contrast with non-speaking role. In Indian film industry a person/organization engaged in the services of providing extras have been classified as 'suppliers'.

Extreme Close-up. (ECU). A strong emphasis shot. A shot in which the subject is much larger than the frame. Provides more detail than a close-up. The abbreviation ECU is often used in a slug line.

Eyelight. A small barndoored or snooted spotlight mounted on or near the camera to give sparkle to the eyes and teeth of a subject.

F

Fade. (Fade to Black, Fade in, Fade out). A smooth, gradual transition from a normal image to complete blackness (Fade out), or vice versa (fade in). An optical effect used as a transitional device.

False Start. When something goes wrong in the film-scene being taken just after it has begun to indicate that the new slate and scene numbers are not needed director/ asst. director calls out 'False start'.

Fast Motion (Skip Frame). A shot in which time appears to move more quickly than normal. The process is commonly achieved by either deleting select frames (called 'skip frames') or be undercranking. See also Frame rate, Judder)

Feature Film. (Feature). A movie at least 60 minutes long intended for theatrical release. A full-length film which is usually fictional.

Feature Presentation. (Main attraction). The main or advertised/declared movie during a screening session.

Federation Internationale Des Archives De Film (FIFA). The International Federation of Film Archives created in Paris in 1938. Most of the National Film Archieves world-over are the affiliated or members of FIFA.

Federation Internationale de la Presse Cinematographique. (FIPRESCI). International Federation of Film Critics.

Federation Internationale des Associations de Producteurs de Film (FIAPF) International Federation of Film Producers Association.

Federation of Film Societies. (FFS). This Indian Film Federation founded in 1960 negotiates concessions from Government of India, obtains films from various countries, issues an occasional journal on Indian-based film culture and is affiliated to International Federation of Film Societies. Celebrated film personality like Satyajit Ray had been president of this Federation in late 40s.

Feedback. In film-sound recording, the return to the input of a part of the output of a machine, system or process.

Famme Fatale. (Literally: 'Deadly Lady'). A slang term used to describe a character in a movie.

Festival of Films. The first film festival took place in Venice (1932). A term 'festival' applies to an event at which films can often premiere Festivals are ordinarily organised for the general film-goers where the participation of experts in the line is solicited. In several countries the film festivals are organized by Government and industry people. Festivals can be used as by studios to show their wares and sell rights to distributors, or to officially mark a movie's release so as to make it eligible for award ceremonies with hard deadlines that can not be met if they waited for a general release. Some festivals are competitive giving awards from a jury or selected by the audiences. In India the Grand Prix — the Golden Peacock —the coveted prize for the best feature film entered in the international film is awarded ceremonially. During the third international and first competitive Film Festival of India (1965) Golden Peacock was awarded to the Sinhalese film 'Gamperaliya' directed by Lester James Peries. That year the jury was headed by Satyajit Ray.

Festival of Films (Indian) Rules for—

While holding this competition in 1965, the following rules were framed. There has been slight modifications during the first three decades.

Except when otherwise provided by the Committee, films entered should: (i) have been produced after January 1, 1963; (ii) Not have been shown in India, except in the case of Indian films; (iii) Not have been entered in any competitive International Film Festival, and (iv) Be consistent with the objectives of the Festival.

The objectives of the Festival are (a) to provide a forum for the participating countries to present films of artistic and cultural value and a high technical standard (b) to contribute to the development of motion picture art and technique; and (c) to promote better understanding between peoples through mutual knowledge and appreciation of good films.

Each country can enter:— One long feature film & one short film. In case a particular country prefers not to enter a long film, it can enter two short films. Except when otherwise provided, short films should not exceed 1500 metres in length. Only films in 35 mm size will be eligible for participation. All films must be shown in their origin languages. Films in language other than English and Hindi must have sub-titles in English or Hindi.

The Jury of long films shall consist of upto 15 Indian or foreign personalities. The Jury of short films shall consist of 5 Indian or foreign personalities. The majority of the Jury members will be non-Indians. At least 1/5th of Jury members shall consist of active film producers.

The votes of the members of the Jury will be by secret ballot. Decisions of the Jury shall be taken by majority of the members voting at the first three ballots and by a relative majority at the fourth ballot, if any, is taken.

The Director of the Festival may be present at the deliberations of the Jury. He will, however, not take part in the vote. No person having participated in the production or distribution of a film shown at the Festival may be a member of the Jury.

The Jury of Long film shall grant: The Golden Award of the International Film Festival of India for the best picture. In addition the Jury may grant: The Jury Special Prize reserved either for a documentary or for another feature film of exceptional quality. The prize for the Best Females acting; the prize for the Best Male acting. Two other prizes to be decided upon by Jury.

The Jury of short films shall grant: The Golden Award of the International Film Festival of India for the best short film.

In addition, the Jury may grant:

Two other prizes which may be decided upon by the Jury. Journalists who are members of the Festival Jury may not send critical reviews of the films submitted to their judgement to newspapers before publication of the Jury's decision.

Festival's Film Symposiums. As part of the Festival, symposiums on the subject relating to the films are also organised. The following foreign specialists had actively participated in the first symposium: Horacio Larreta (Argentina), Mr. Erich Svabik (Czechoslovakia), Axel Jepsen (Denmark), Aito Nakinen (Finland), Georges Sadoul (France), Guilio Casare Castello (Italy), Masayoshi Iwabutchi (Japan), Boleslaw Michalech (Poland), Idestam Almcuist (Sweden), Dr. Roger Manvell (U.K.) & Marie Seton (U.K.).

Festschrift. A festival publication of books/films. A publication of book is commonly a collection of experts. These publications are mostly priced publications and serve the purpose of souvenir.

Fesse. (Also Fess) film. A film rated as 'ordinary'.

Filius nalluis film. The success of a film is shared by everybody that works for the production of the film. However, the failure is not claimed by anybody. In such cases that film is the product of nobody.

Fill light. A light used to fill in shadow cast by the key light and thus balance the picture.

Film Advisory Board. In India in June 1940 an advising body was set up to advice the then Government of India on the production and distribution of films on war propaganda.

Film Abstract. Variety of experimental films of a non-figurative nature are called as abstract films. The abstract film had its origins in the *avant-Grade* movements of the twenties. These abstract films were of two types viz. depicting photographic reality and graphic material. Viking Eggeling and Hans Richter are recognized as pioneers of abstract films of scroll drawing (1918-1920). Both in photographic and animation forms of the abstract films, visual interpretations of music became a particular manifestation. The painter Marcel Duchamp achieved for the first time in giving 3-dimensional effect by using motorized optical devices in his abstract film (Cinema Anemic' which he produced in collaboration with Man Ray and Mare Allegret (1926).

Film & Television Studies. Numerous Institutes and organizations in India and abroad have prepared systematic studies in the various branches of film and television faculty. These subjects are also taught on the university level. There are very many universities which are imparting film and television training. American studies at Brunel University at Uxbridge UB8 3PH, United Kingdom is one of the most reputed universities which through its Faculty of Arts plays an important role to provide support to the aspirants by developing their academic interests and exploring new areas. This faculty offers an enriching and stimulating learning environment for each student who chooses to join them. Details and the film and television studies of Brunnel University are available from its Faculty of Arts located at Uxbridge UB8, 3PH or/and from British Councils' libraries established in different parts of the world. At present modules in film and television studies of Brunnel's are one of the following 3 levels:

Level 1: Introduction to Film & Television, Audio Visual Theory and Practice, Critical Methodologies. The Developing of the Moving Image, A Case Study of British Film and Television in the 1960s.

Level 2: Video Production, Television Forms and Meaning, Science Fictions, New Hollywood Cinema, Theory & Practice of Photography (for single honours students only), European Cinema, British Film & Television, Melodrama: A Thematic Study, Hong Kong Cinema.

Level 3: Documentary: Theory & Practice, Special Project (Dissertation), Activism and Television, Gender and Sexuality, Third Cinema, Psychoanalysis and the Moving Image, The Horror Film, Comedy, Death and the Moving Image.

Film Bin. Large receptable in which film is allowed to fall while assembling shots or when running film through a viewer or projector.

Film Buyer. A person who arranges to purchase films from a distributor on behalf of an exhibitor.

Film Cement. Liquid used for joining pieces of film.

Film Commissions. These commissions assist film industry in finding locations for the proposed films. These are also assisting in planning a production which involves a local, over night, or distant location shoot.

Film Conversation Tables. Between the picture and the sound that corresponds to it, there is a 20 frame separation on the 35 mm film and 26 frame separation on 16mm film as the sound head of the projection is that distance from the light separation through which the picture is projected on the screen.

Film Daily Year Book. (FDY Book). United Trades' Annual devoted to films. First published in 1918 and the publication was suspended in the year 1971. The year book covered the vital information on all the aspects of movies produced in the previous year and used to provide statistical data. Mr. B.V. Dharap — Indian Film-Historian - has brought out such Film Annuals during 60s and 70s, and these publication activities were stopped suddenly after his sad demise.

Film Developing. (Developed). A process whereby images recorded on film stock are transferred to a negative print. See also colour timing.

Film Exposing. In the movie-camera the film is stored in light-tight boxes, from which it is drawn by means of a sprocket or toothed when engages in the film perforations. It then moves intermittently pass the camera gate — the spot in camera where the film reaches the aperture through which it will be exposed, or the point where the image formed by the lens is focussed upon the sensitive surface. The image is recorded while the film is stationary, and it only moves down when a revolving-disc shutter, which is linked to the transit mechanism, momentarily obscures the lens. After exposure the film is wound into a second light-tight box.

Film Festivals. Please see 'Festival of Films' and also Festival of Films (Indian) Rules for.

Film Finance Corporation. (FFC). Recognising the immediate need to encourage film of high aesthetic standards, Government of India established in Film Finance Corporation (FFC). FFC extends loans and facilities to talented young film-makers. FFC is also involved in importing films from many parts of the world.

Film Formula. A term refers to emotion and suspense in films.

Film Grain. (Grain, Graininess, Grainy). The tiny particles of light-sensitive material on film stock that record images. Finer grains give higher image quality, but coarser grains allow a faster shutter speed. Grainness is an artifact which results from the use of coarse grains, and gives image a slight mosaic appearance.

Film Institute of India. (FII). Later Film & T.V. Institute of India (FTII) FII was set up on the recommendations of the Film Enquiry Committee Report of 1951. On December 27, 1959 the Prabhat Film Studio, Pune was acquired by the Government of India to set up this film institute. The regular courses of FTI started in 1961. Within three decades of its inception FTI switched over to accommodate television courses along with others and by this time acquired a spacious residential campus for its students, its own processing laboratory, 3 studio floors, 16 stand-back editing tables, a ready army of 16 mm and 35 mm film-cameras, extensive video shooting and editing facilities and 3 viewing theatres.

Prof. John Caroll from the Australian National Film & T.V. school assisted FTII as a fresh curriculum designer consultant in early January 2000. He helped FTII in designing its new courses and felt that digital technology was the future. Accordingly a new course has been introduced by FTII which will cater to digital production and post-production requirements.

Film Magazines. 1. Monthly periodicals/programmes on the interests which are devoted to the subject of films. 2. A reel of film-stock ready for use in a camera. The clapper-loader is responsible for inserting these into a camera.

Film-makers. A collective term used to refer to people who have a significant degree of control over the creation and making of a movie. Directors, producers, screenwriters and editors are these main exponents of the team.

Film-making, Methods of. It has been found that there are 3 main methods of filming and film-making. These methods are as follows: (i) first the picture is taken on the 35 mm, negative and positive release prints are made from it either in 35 mm or 16 mm. width. (ii) The picture is photographed on 16 mm. Negative and release prints are made on 16 mm. positive (iii) The picture is photographed on 16 mm. reversal film. This is the method used for 'home movies' when only one print of the picture is needed.

Any picture made in 35 mm. width can be successfully reduced to the 16 mm. width. In India sporadic efforts have been made by regional languages' film-makers to enlarge to 16mm. Film to the 35mm. width, but these films were not accepted by the viewers and as such these have not proved to be successful at the box office.

Filmology. The study or/and analysis of the technological, social, economic, political and historical nature of film as a phenomenon of cause and effect.

Film Noir. (Black film). Describes a genre of film which typically features dark, brooding characters, corruption, detectives and the seedy side of the big city.

Films, Objectionable. Almost all the countries have shown their likes/dislikes as regards to the films that are screened. Till early 60s, in Indian film-making the following subjects were treated as objectionable subjects for showing them on the screen. With the growing influence of western films and likes, a dislikes of Indian cinegoers these have been more or less modified adequately to the present period. However, the spirit behind making these rules remains the same as before. Ordinarily, the following kinds of films are liable to objection:

- Extreme crime or which familiarise young people with crime so as to make them conclude that theft, robbery and crimes of violence are normal incidents of ordinary day-to-day life and not greatly to be reprobated, or which exhibit the actual methods by which thieves carry out their purpose and make the methods of crime the chief theme, or in which crime is the dominant feature of a serial and not merelv an episode in the story.
- Undermine the teaching of morality by showing vice in attractive form even though retribution follows, or casting a halo of glory or success round the heads of the vicious, or suggesting that a person is morally justified in succumbing to temptation in order to escape from bad circumstances or uncongenial work, or bringing into contempt the institution of marriage or suggesting abnormal sexual relations, or lowering the sacredness of the family ties.
- Exhibit indecorous dress or absolute nudity of the living (except infants and small children) or nude statues of figures in suggestive positions.
- Bring into contempt public characters acting as such e.g. ministers of religion, ambassadors and official representatives of foreign nation, judges, the police, civil servants of Government, etc.
- Are calculated to wound the susceptibilities of foreign nations or of members of any religion.
- Are calculated or possibly intended to format social unrest and discontent, i.e. not scenes merely depicting realistically the hard conditions under which people live, but depicting the violence that results in an actual conflict between Capital and Labour.
- Are calculated to promote disaffection or resistance to Government or to promote a breach of law and order.

Films. Objectionable subject of— Soon after the Indian Independence years, certain rules and regulation were laid down for the execution of Central Board of Film Censors. Earlier to that during the British regime provincial censorship of films had been in force and the objectionable subjects were notified. In Mumbai (then Bombay), the Bombay Board of Film Censors was first constituted in 1920. There were 6 members, 3 of whom were non-officials representing the Hindu, Muslim and Parsee communities. The Commissioner of Police was the ex-official President of the Board. There were 2 inspectors under the Board. In Punjab, Board of Film Censors was first constituted in 1927 and there were 12 members. In Bengal, the Board was first constituted in 1920. In Chennai (then Madras) the Board was first constituted in June 1920, and there were 19 members.

Before Independence in India the main responsibility of the Censor Board was to ensure that the rulers were not shown in an adverse light, and the political status and dignity was maintained. After 1947, the emphasis shifted the morality, mainly to sex and in a feeble sort of way towards violence. Till early 60s, in Indian film-making, the following subjects were treated as objectionable subjects. With the spreading influence of western films and likes and dislikes of Indian film-viewers there have been more or less modified rules adequate to the present period. However, the spirit behind making these rules remains to be the same as before.

The following is a list of film-subjects which was then considered as 'likely to be objectionable':

- Indecorous, ambiguous or irreverent titles and subjects.
- The irreverent treatment or sacred subjects.

- Materialisation of the conventional figure of any founder of religion.
- Excessively passionate love scenes.
- Indelicate sexual situations.
- Scenes suggestive of immorality.
- Men and women in bed together.
- Situations accentuating delicate marital relations.
- 'First Night' scenes.
- Confinements.
- Subjects dealing with the premeditated seduction of girls.
- Scenes depicting the effect of venereal diseases, inherited or acquired.
- Subjects dealing with the 'white colour slave' traffic.
- Scenes laid in brothels.
- Prostitution and procuration.
- Illicit sexual relationship.
- Incidents suggestive of incestuous relations.
- Themes and reference related to 'race suicide'.
- Incidents which indicated the actual perpetration of criminal assaults on women.
- Nude figures.
- Unnecessary exhibition of feminine under-clothing.
- Bathing scenes passing the limits of propriety.
- Indecorous dancing.
- Offensive vulgarity and impropriety in conduct or dress.
- Vulgar accessories in the staging.

- Cruelty to young infants and excessive cruelty and torture to adults, especially women.
- Cruelty to animals.
- Cruelsome murders and strangulation scenes.
- Execution.
- The modus operandi of criminals.
- Drunken scenes carried to excess.
- The drug habit, e.g. opium, morphia, cocaine, wine etc.
- References to controversial politics.
- Relations of capital and labour.
- Scenes tending to disparage public characters and institutions.
- Scenes holding up the national flag to contempt or ridicule.
- Subjects dealing with India, attempting to suggest the disloyalty of Government servants or bringing into dispute the Government prestige.
- The exhibition of profuse bleeding.
- Realistic horrors of warfare.
- Scenes and incidents calculated in time or war to afford information to the enemy.
- The exploitation of tragic incidence of the war.
- Incidents having a tendency to disparage other nations.
- Brutal fighting.
- References to illegal operations.
- Intimate biological studies unsuitable for general exhibition.
- Gross stavesties of the administration of justice.
- Serving and drinking liquors.

- Blackmail associated with immorality.
- Companionate marriage and free love.
- Unrelieved sordid themes.
- Unpleasant details of medical operations.

Film piracy. The crime of dealing with the business of selling films, videos etc. making infringement of copyright. An act of handling films/film business without proper authority. Running unlicensed film business.

Film, Pornographic. *See* Pornographic Film.

Film, Printer. Printers intended for large quantity of work are of the contact type. But for special work optical type of printers are used. These are similar in principal to enlarger or projection printer, the two films being separated, with a lens system, between the two films moving in opposite directions. The projection printer is used to introduce effects such as fading, wipes and multiple exposures from the normal negatives which have been obtained in the camera. A duplicate negative is prepared from the original 'master positive' thus obtained, and from this, further soft positive, which in their turn yield the negatives which are used for making the large quantities of prints which are actually used in the cinemas.

Film Printing. The process of transferring images from a negative print to a print. A roll of finished negative and the roll of unexposed positive film are loaded into a machine, and past together past a printing point behind which a light is situated. Thus light can be controlled in intensity to compensate for differences in sensitive negative density. There are two kinds of printer: (i) The intermittent in which the negative and positive, inclose contact, pause in the printing gate while the exposure is made, and (ii) the continuous type of printer where the pair of films runs smoothly past a printing slit.

Film Projecting. The picture projects is similar in principle in camera, except that the film is moved past the picture aperture by means of an intermittent sprocket, or 'Maltse Cross' movement, instead of a claw mechanism. In this illumination is provided by a light of high density used in conjunction with a condenser, but only the picture portion is projected on to the cine screen.

Film Punctuations, Standard Methods of—

(i) By direct cut. In this method one shot immediately succeeds the next. Impressions: speed. If well done, clean and sense of restlessness and jerky continuity. (ii) By fade in and fade-out. The gradual emergence of a shot from a black frame, and its opposite. (iii) By dissolve. The gradual change in one scene to another by superimposition of the images, the end of the first shot being carefully timed in relation to the emergence of the next. (iv) By applying wipe. The effect of the wipe has been described as if an invisible roller were passed over the screen horizontally or vertically, wiping out one picture and revealing the next. (v) By continuity title. Words cease on the sound track and either silence or music ensues. (vi) By other camera devices. Not involving a cut, dissolve or fade.

Film Quarterly. United States' Journal erstwhile *Hollywood Quarterly* (1945) is being published by California Press.

Film Society. The first group of its kind in the world was founded in London in 1925 to promote the intellectual respectability of the cinema by showing the important and influential films denied commercial exhibition. Founder members of this Film Society were literature-wizards like H.G. Wells and George Bernard Shaw. The last of the Society's 108 programmes was presented on April 23, 1939.

Film Shot is cinematic way of stating movement. It is also a way of camera to handle movement. Establishing, explanatory and climatic are the three kinds of groups formed in the film shot process.

Film Shots. (Censored). Film censor is an agent of the Government in most of the countries and sex, violent crime, politics etc. have been the sensitive topics in the jurisdiction of sensors. Penal of the Central Board of Film Censors in India within the frame-work and guiding principles decide the suitability of the film for exhibition. (refer to 'Objectionable Films).

Kobita Sarkar, authors of 'Indian Cinema Today" and "You Can't Please Everyone" was Member of the Advisory Panel of the Central Board of Film Censors in Bombay and Calcutta during the period 1964 and 1977. She has quoted several pertinent examples of censored film shots in her book "You can't please everyone" both from foreign and Indian Films which have had come for scrutiny. The following selected censored film cases are quoted from that book.

'Rose Tattoo' had one deletion which read: Alvaro saying, "He chased my grandmother in a flooded rice field, she slip on a wet rock-Here I am."

From 'Carpetbeggers' the dialogues considered highly reprehensible:

Cord: A man is judged by what's in his head, not in his bed.

Jonas: You dried up important old man.

Similarly quite a few selected examples from Indian regional films: From a Hindi film 'Main Hoon Alladin' a deletion in Reel III which goes as follows:

In a dance sequence, shots of the prominent views of the dancers waving their hips indecorously. In a Tamil Film, Panam Padaithavan Reel 6, Cabaret Dance. Delete (a) Close shot of dancer rolling her abdomen in a vulgar fashion. (b) jerking her loins (c) her stripping clothes and (d) her waist dance. Delete the 8 inserts of the half-naked second cabaret dancer. In Kaliyodom, a Malayalam film, 'the kissing gesture of the bride and bridegroom had to go.' In a Telgu film, Devata', in Reel 4. 'In the dance-song delete the dancer violently tilting her breasts, stretching her legs sideways when the undergarments are seen in silhouette.'

Film Stock. The physical medium on which photographic images are recorded.

Film Story, Picture. "The Great Train Robbery (1906) is recognised as having a complete story. It was 800 ft. in length and was based on cinematic actions.

Film Strip. This term refers to still pictures printed in sequence on a strip film. The film-strip provides the simplest, most direct, and least expensive mass medium of communication. The film-strip came into being shortly before 1920 when Underwoods of New York conceived the idea of putting their large photographic library on 55mm film. Later 35 mm film was found more desirable and became the standard width for the film strip. The single frame film strip is run through the projector vertically.

Film tricks. The name of M. Melies who made "Cinderalla" "Red Riding Hood" and "A Trip to the Moon" is considered as the Father of the Film tricks. Mr. D.G. Phalke—father of the Indian Films—who made the Indian film possible and sowed the seed of this great industry was the first film-maker in India to show film-tricks in his silent movies. Though several stalwarts in the film industry have had effectively used this device of film tricks in their films, Babubhai Mistry's name is considered as Guru of Hindi films' film tricks, as he had mastered this device with his unique skills of presentation on the screen.

Film, Underground. See 'Underground film'.

Film Viewer. Hand operated or motor driven machine providing a small moving picture when film is drawn through its useful for viewing film material during editing. In film viewer, the film is drawn through the machine and magnified picture appears on a ground glass screen.

Filmology. The study or/and analysis of the technological, social, economic, political and historical nature of film as phenomenon of cause and effect.

Films Division. (FD). The division (branch) of the Ministry of Information and Broadcasting was set up in 1948, with headquarters in Mumbai (then Bombay). Documentary films produced by F.D. are called Documentary films of Indian while the newsreels are named Indian News Review. FD is the single largest producer of documentaries all over the world.

Films, Duplicating. In the production process of motion pictures, duplication stages are frequently employed for various reasons. For example, duplication is used wherever effects such as Lap dissolves, fades, wipes blow-ups of a portion of the original scene etc. are to be introduced. These effects are prepared by making a master positive from the original negative, using an optical printer. A duplicate negative is then made from the master positive for use in making the release print. In general, wherever optical printing is called for duplication is required.

Films. Export of. See Export of Films.

Films & Filming. A monthly publication published by Hansom Books, London. Considered as one of the standard and authoritative publication on the subject of films and filming.

Films Purpose of. See Purpose of films.

Films, Storage of. Since Cine films are subject to changes in their physical and photographic properties like any other stored sensitized material it becomes very much essential to create storage conditions which will ensure that these changes are kept to a minimum, in order to maintain uniform results in processing. Although cine films are only made on safety base, when choosing or constructing a film store it must be remembered that old films or nitrate base or spools with pliced-in-replacement on nitrate base, will continue to be encountered for years together. As long as it is possible that there are part of entire spools on nitrate base in the store, the great danger of easy inflammability inherent in nitrate film will endanger the entire store. In almost every country in the world, the storage of nitrate films is governed by stringent safety regulations which must be adhered to strictly concerning the equipment and maintenance of such place. Premises housing such stores should be constructed of fire-proof material and fire extinguishers and air-conditioning plant must be provided. The air conditioning plant must be installed in such a way that the highly poisonous gases, generated by burning nitrate film, can be diverted to the outside air thus preventing them penetrating into other parts of the building. Besides adequate fire-prevention care must also be taken to avoid damage of water. In case of raw films' storage two different stores i.e. one for safety film and one for nitrate film are established. For satisfactory climatic conditions 18°C (65°F) and a relative humidity of the air up to 70% is recommended for storage upto a maximum period of six months.

Films, Statutory Indian Film Societies. The credit for pioneering Indian film society belongs to Mumbai (then Bombay) and Calcutta film societies. Long before moving into the film-making, celebrated film-director Satyajit Ray founded the Calcutta Film Society. Quite a few Indian film societies are regularly functioning in the proper perspective. The Anandam Film Society in Mumbai is still a leading one in these series. Gopal Dutia's yeomen service and contribution to the film society will always be remembered. The Film Cultural

Centre in Pune founded by B.J. Nag and G. Mahambare in 1961 organised for some time important and significant activities under the patronage and active support of veteran film actor Gajanan Jagirdar. Ashay Film Club running on the same lines from Pune and Prabhat Mitra Mandal, Mumbai are presently doing very remarkable work in this field.

Final cut. (In editing). The polished completed work print.

Final mix. The combination of various sound-tracks into one composite master, often after the intermediate stage of pre-mixing.

Flashback. A scene in the film that breaks the chronological continuity of the main narrative by depicting image/ events that have happened in the past. This is in contrast with the flashforward.

Flashforward. A scene that breaks the continuity which is chronological in order of the main narrative in the film. It depicts events which happen in the future. This is contrast with flashback — the term explained above.

Flashing. The laboratory technique of exposing film to a very low level of illumination.

Flat. A wooden frame-work supporting stretched and painted cloth used as a background of action while filming.

Flatbed Editing Machine. A machine where the positive rolls of the film sound, music, and effects tracks are placed flat as on a table.

Fliers. Economical leaflets advertising a film that is under production or already completed and ready for screening.

Foam Technician. (Foam Runner). A person from the team of film-making who is responsible for creating foam latex prosthetic appliances from a sculpture created by a make-up artists.

Focal Press. The world-known Publishers of communication techniques' books. Focal Press is an imprint of the Butterworth Group which has brought out numerous publications on the various aspects of film and filming. A number of books are being printed and added to these useful collection.

Focus. The sharpness of an image, or the adjustments made on a camera necessary to achieve this. A point at which rays that is of light, heat or sound coverage or from which they appear to diverge after reflection or refraction.

Focus Group. A group of approximately 10 to 12 members of the public, unrelated to a movie's production who attend a sneak preview. A single focus group is ordinarily composed of a selection within the boundaries of a movie's intended audience. The group is extensively questioned by the film-makers following the screening. The opinions expressed by the focus group are incorporated into any further editing that may occur before the premiers of the film.

Focus Puller. A member of the camera crew who adjusts the focus of the camera during filming.

Fog level. The photographic density of the unexposed film after development.

Foley. The art of creating incidental effects such as footsteps and movement in synchronization with the visual component of a movie. Named after an early practitioner Foley artists sometimes use bizarre objects and methods to achieve sound effects. These sounds are very often exaggerated for extra-effect for fight sequence etc.

Foley Artist. (Foley Operator). A person in the team who creates foley sound effects. Mr. Kamat was known as an foley artist in the Indian Hindi Films during early 50s, and new versatile artists have since entered this line.

Foley Editor. A person in the team who edits the sounds created by a foley artist.

Foley Mixer. A person in a team who is specialized in sound mixing and who works closely with a foley artist to record sound effects.

Follow action. (follow-shot). The camera moves horizontally or vertically on its tripod or on a dolly in such a manner as to keep constant attention centred on key action.

Footage Counter. The device which is having numbers to indicate the footage from start mark of a reel of a film being shooted.

Four-walling. Renting an individual theatre for a very short period for the purpose of exhibiting films.

Frame. An individual picture image which eventually appears on a print.

Frame line. The line (narrow) or area between the frames.

Frame Rate. (Frames per second. FPS). Movies are created by taking a rapid sequence of pictures (frames) of action. By displaying these frames at the same rate at which they were recorded, the illusion of motion can be created. 'Frame rate' is the number of frames captured or projected per second. The human optical system is only capable of capturing pictures 18-20 times per second; hence to give a realistic illusion of motion a frame rate which is greater than this is required. Most modern pictures are filmed and displayed at 24 frames per second. Earlier films used lower frame rates and hence when they were played back on the modern equipment, fast motion occurs due to undercranking.

Frame. Zero. Refer to the term Zero Frame.

Free Cinema. (1956-59). The film movement activated by Anderson, Reisz, Lassally, Fletcher et al to revolt against orthodoxy in literature and theatre through the film medium.

Free Clicks. In music clicks heard by the musicians that a set tempo and are not included as part of the score.

Free Timing. Music recorded to clock or film without benefit of clicks.

Freeze Frame. (Freezes). An optical printing effect whereby a single frame is repeated to give the illusion that all action has stopped. Often used by Martin Scorsese. A term Freeze/frame is in contrast with stop motion.

Freeze shot. Pertains to the technique used in slide motion films.

French scene. A dramatic unit under the system of designation which decrees a new scene to begin with each other non-incidental entrance or exit.

Friese Greene's Invention. Camera is an apparatus for throwing an image of an object through a lens upon a screen, for the purpose of drawing, instruction or photographic record. For the first-named purposes it was called the camera obscure, having its modern outcome in the periscope. Thomas Wedgwood utilized the camera for developed type of photography before 1802 and the same technique was in vogue for some time. William Friese-Green is the first technician who invented moving picture camera. He was the father of the movie camera and all the relevant cinematic developments in cine-photography are based on his invention.

Front Lighting. General flat and featureless lighting that emanates from the camera area or front of a set.

Frozen work print. The definitive version of the image as they will be seen in the finished picture.

Full animation. A term used to denote movement of everything in picture, frame by frame, in cartoon subjects. This method is supposed to be most costly of all the animation methods.

Full coat. A 35 mm film covered with a magnetic coating ready for use for recording.

Fullscreen (4:3). This term is used to describe the shape of the picture a movie is displayed in order for it to fill a regular (as of 1998) Television screen. (Aspect ratio 4:3)

Full shot. A shot that takes in all of a subject; be it an individual, a group, a car or a house.

Fusion. (As in Music). 1. A close union of things, as if melted together. 2. Coalition.

Futze. (In sound recording). The quality added to sound that coming over a radio or telephone.

G

G (General). A certificate issued by the MPAA indicating that a film in question in suitable for all ages.

Gaffar. (Chief Lighting Technician). The need of the electrical and lighting department. In early modern English this term is meant 'old man'. Named after the gaffing hook which manipulates the overhead hanging lights.

Gamma. The degree of contrast in a negative or a print.

Gang Swing. Please refer to Swing, Gang.

Garden hose pan. When the camera turns to left or right, then it returns to former position.

Gasper colour. Colour print process developed in England. Named after Bela Gaspar (1934).

Gate. A section in a camera or projector mechanism where the film passes behind the lens.

Gauge. A convenient and commodious reference to film size by measurement of its width.

Gemini System. Method of linking of 16 mm film to a television camera.

Gimmic. 1. Any secret device for performing a trick. 2. In film-story writing or script writing, a clever plot device, especially one that helps to resolve the film's problem.

Glass shot. Scene shot through optical shot on which part of a scene is painted to achieve a special effect. In contrast with the term 'process shot' involving rear projection.

Gobo. A term refers to the portable, light deflecting or sound-absorbing panel mounted on an adjustable stand which can be raised or lowered. A small gobo is called a 'flag.'

Go-Motion. (Go Motion). A form of animation similar to stop motion. But go-motuon incorporates motion blur. Ordinary stop motion can not produce motion blur as motion only occurs between the frames. Robotic models that are moved during the exposure of each frame produce motion blur, and thus they are more realistic. Go-motion has been pioneered by Industrial Light and Magic for 'Dragonslayer' a film released in 1981. Dragonslayer — a dark ages fairy tale — was directed by Matthew Robbins in which young Peter MacNicol played a sorcerer's apprentice who is called upon to slay a fearsome flying dragon. The super special effects employed in this film were claimed as the 'real stars' because "when the huge, fire-breathing dragon goes into action, the film-story came alive." (Critic's review).

Gradation. The variation in tonal values in a photographic image.

Grainness. In sound recording it is very obviously important that fluctuations in the sources of illumination used for recording and printing shall be prevented, and that all causes of non-uniformity in development be minimized. However, when all these are done there are still variations in the capacity of exposed film. These variations are usually referred to as 'grainness'.

Grammy Awards. In Music, these are annually awarded to the best song, best rock song, best make rock vocal performance are best song written for a movie or television. One of such songs is selected as the Music Record of the Year and also the other one as Best Album of the Year.

Grey Wedge. Also known as 'Density wedge'. Strip of transparent material increasing in density from one end to another. Moved along in front of the lens, it gradually decreases or increases the amount of light reaching the film. Used for fades.

Greensman. A member of the crew who procures, places, and maintains any vegetation on a set.

Grid. Network of conductors for distribution of electric power.

Grip. In the United Kingdom, a grip is a person who works exclusively with equipment that the camera is mounted on. While in the United States of America, a grip is a person who is responsible for the adjustment and maintenance of production equipment on the set. Their typical duties include laying dolly tracks or erecting scaffolding.

Ground Glass. In cine-photography, optically ground glass through which cameraman looks to correct focus of lens.

Ground Noise Reduction. During the times of low modulation that noise is most objectionable. For this, ground-noise, reduction systems are used. These systems are used for variable-area recording provide for making off the unused portion of a sound track area. This may be done by biasing the galvanometer, or by use of a shutter whose vanes cut off a portion of the recording beam during the periods of low modulation. The shutter vanes move relatively slowly in and out, following the envelop of the waves recorded by the galvanometer. In variable-density systems ground noise reduction takes the form of making the prints darker at times of low modulation. In light valve systems this is accomplished by bringing the ribbons of the light valves closer together by means of abusing current while in the penumbra system of variable-density recording, using the galvanometer a separate electromagnetic device similar to the shutter used for variable-area recording moves the vane, the shadow of whose edge constitutes the penumbra.

Gyro Head. A camera mounting on tripod or dolly, which enables the operator to move the camera smoothly and quickly to any desire direction.

Guide Track. A sound track taped on location for later use to synchronize sound in looping and dubbing session.

Gutta-percha. A tough plastic substance obtained from the latex of serial several Malaysian trees and used especially for electric insulation.

H

Hair-light. A separate light that strikes the subject from behind and overhead, creating an effect on the head and shoulders.

Hair stylist. Person responsible for maintaining actors' hairstyles during filming. Hair stylists are also known as Hair dressers.

Halation. Salo surrounding true image of films. Caused by light too bright on the subject.

Halation by Irradiation. While considering the physical properties of Agfa-Black & White and Colour films, during exposure, part of the light reaching the emulsion layer of the film is absorbed and usefully employed by the light-sensitive silver halide crystals contained in the emulsion to form the picture. A small amount of light is reflected by the sliver bromide crystals dispersed within the emulsion and can thus create the effect known as 'Halation by irradiation!

Halogen Light, Tungsten. Please see Tungsten Halogen light,

Handheld. Footage shot with the camera placed on the cameraman's shoulder or in his her hands instead of on a tripod/dolly.

Hardtop. A slang for a normal indoor theatre.

Harmonizer. Electronic device which can correct out-of-pitch singing.

Hat light. A special light used in older films to fill in the shadow cast by the brim (margin) of a performer's hat.

Hays Production Code. (Hays Code, Hays Office, Hays Production Office). Named after Will H. Hays (1879-1954) who was Postmaster General under the Republican President Warren Harding. In the 1920s, the American film-goers became alarmed at the increasingly frequent portrayal of violence, sex and lawlessness on the movie screens to avoid troublesome government regulation, the then Motion Picture Producers of America created their own regulatory body and appointed W.H. Hays as Head. His influence became so great that the body became known as 'Hays Office'. The Hays Production Code for Motion Pictures was introduced in 1934. Films such as "Who's Afraid of Virginia Woolf?" based on the famous Edward Albee play (1966) and "Blow-up" — a fascinating and thought-provoking drama involving a London photographer who believes he has witnessed a murder (1966) inspire MPAA President Jack Valenti to abolish the Hays Code as his first step in overhauling the certificate system in 1967.

Head. The start or front of a roll of a film.

Head on shot Movement. Straight into a camera, as in the case of someone striding down a hall.

Head-on and Trail-away. Arrangement of shot which marks the removal of a character from the stage of our attention.

Heavy Role. A villain-type of character.

High angle shot. Shot taken looking down on the subject.

High frequency Losses. Much of the progress towards the better sound quality has been in the removal of some of the limiting factors that so restricted the frequency range in the earlier sound records, making them muffled and hard to understand. Now-a-days most of the improvement is possible due to the availability of better optical systems, narrower recording slits, finer grain films, ultraviolet light recording and printing, lens surface treatment to reduce reflection and control of processing besides all the latest technical amenities. Literature on the subject of processing for improved high frequency is rare in density recording contrary to the area of recording as in the case of area recording sporadic factors largely dictate exposures and developments for both negatives and prints. In area systems, satisfying the cross-modulation tests, while not guaranteeing good high frequency responses, never conflicts.

High-frequency Losses, Compensation of. In sound recording this practice was adopted in the beginning for the expected high frequency loss by exaggeration process. Since the new and recent developments in this field it is not now necessary to make excessively large allowance for expected high frequency loss.

High Hat. Extremely low camera mount for use on floor or table where tripod would be inconvenient.

High Key. Images that exhibit a tendency to lighter tones. A brilliantly illuminated setting used usually to heighten gaiety of comedies. Low key lighting is used to heighten suspense or for heavy dramas.

Highlight. The brightest lit and lightest coloured points of a subject.

Hold. A word used in a continuity report to indicate that a particular take should be kept, but not developed.

Holes, Sprocket. Please refer to Sprocket Holes.

Hollywood. California's (U.S.) Hollywood is famous as the centre of the U.S. Motion picture industry. A film-style characterized by professionalism, dramatic realism, pace, a straight forward narrative mode and usually a star name have been the main features. Many film artists from world over harbour love for making appearance in Hollywood films. There have been few movies depicting the Hollywood life. In 'Hollywood Canteen' produced in 1944. Director Delmer Daves has had been successful in presenting a galaxy of Hollywood star who made their guest appearances in the film. This film was then acclaimed as the "review of the entertainment community's supporting efforts during World War II". "Hollywood Boulevard (1977)" and "The Hollywood Knights (1980)" had proved to be successful at the box office Honey Wagon. A *trailer* or vehicle that contains restroom facilities and dressing rooms for personnel for use during a location shoot.

Hook. A striking incident, unique action or the like, used to capture attention of the audience at the beginning of the picture. A linking device used to render dialogue cohesive by tying each speech one ahead of it.

Hopalong Cassidy. Between 1935 and 1940, William Boyd (1898-1972) made 26 films based on Clarence E. Mulford's cowboy character. Boyd got international fame for his typical appearance, actions, fighting and characterization in these films.

Hot Mike. A microphone which is on and receiving. It is also called 'Live Mike.'

Hot Set. A set on which a scene is in process of being shot. It is exclusively labelled as 'hot shot' to indicate that it should not be changed or disturbed.

Hot splicer. Also called 'Heat Splicer'. A joiner that incorporates a heating device in the elements.

Hot Spot. Small area of a scene which has been too brightly lighted. A term 'hot spot' also denotes a flare-back into camera from bright metallic or reflecting surfaces.

Hue. The essence of a colour determined by spectral wavelength; chroma, as opposed to value or saturation.

Huston Style. Named after John Huston (born: 1906) U.S. Director who was first Hollywood Director to insist on making films where the stories took place.

Huxley's Biologicals. British biologist Sir Julian Huxley (1887-1975) was the general supervisor of biological films for Gaumont-British Instructional. He framed and maintained certain standards for the purpose of making films having accent on Biology. Later he was able to devise a film series on evolution.

Hype. Overzealous praise or advertising.

Hypersonic. Of a being a speed over five times that of the speed of sound.

I

I.F.I. The Information Films of India (Feb. 1943 - May 1946) (I.F.I.) during the course of 3 years produced 101 shorts, several of which were chosed for exhibition abroad. IFI was abolished in consequence of a cut motion passed by the Indian Legislative Assembly. Besides English, I.F.I. produced documentaries in Bengali, Hindi, Tamil and Telgu languages.

Identification. The tendency of a screen-play's audience to take sides, in effect cheering the hero and booing the villian.

Incident light meter. Exposure meter that indicates the intensity of light falling on a subject.

Inciting action. Also called Exciting Force. An early incident that reveals what the plot is going to be about.

Independent film. (India) A movie not produced by any major studio.

Indian Motion Pictures Export Corporation. (IMPEC). This quasi-Government body has been established in India to streamline exports, avoid under-hand dealing and promote cultural relationship.

Inflactions. In film-music, increases or decreases in volume to effect musical nuances.

Infrared. An invisible form of light that includes heat.

Ink. (Verb). To sign a contract. (Noun) Press Coverage.

Inky Dinky. A 150/200 watt bulb used to highlight certain scenes from the film.

Inking. A period of time.

Insert. In filming, a close-up shot of an object which is produced by the second unit. The term 'insert' probably came about to reflect the fact that this shot taken by the second unit will be 'inserted' into the final version of the movie during editing.

Institut des Hautes Etudes Cinematographiques. (IDHEC) This Institute is formed by the French Government in Paris in 1943 with a dual purpose of training film-makers and developing film-appreciation at all levels. Though there is no script-writers' course at IDHEC, Institute's students are encouraged to write their own film-scripts for their Diploma Courses. Students of all disciplines such as directors, editors, sound operators etc. work together and produce films, conforming to their courses. Film Institute of India (FII) under its first principle-film director-actor Gajanan Jagirdar in its initial stages was affiliated to IDHFC and thereby acquired expertise from this IDHEC. IDHEC's then Director Mr. Remy Tessonnen had then visited Indian Film Institute very often and had fruitful discussions with several Ministry of Information & Broadcasting officials and FII's staff on the proceedings of running film institutes.

Instructional Films. Also called Teaching Films. These are exclusively produced for the purpose of demonstrations. These type of films are made to instruct certain groups with common specialized interests in various professions, faculties, drades or civic activities.

Interent. Film-editing by juxtaposition of elements.

Interior. Indicates that the scene or a shot filmed/to be filmed indoors.

Intermezzo. A short dramatic or musical entertainment as entracts enacted during the film-festivals'/awards-trophies distribution programmes etc. Both famous and budding film artists or/and playback artists participate in such ceremonial programme.

Internate. (Also Internet) The world-wide popular effective medium being used in the various fields of film—making. Internate provides general information on media or entertainment business. It also assists in production-marketing and distribution. It is very much useful in planning of films & film-making and in the process of fund-raising for the scheduled film-production. The websites of different agencies/persons help performing research and developing communication skills with the concerned parties.

Intermediate. A process in the laboratory that is necessary or valuable in proceeding from the original form of material to some required duplicate.

International Film Festivals. Cannes and Venice Film Festivals gave recognition to the cinema as an art medium. First International Film Festival in India was held in 1952.

International Track. In sound recording, a mixed sound track with all the elements except dialogue.

Internet. See 'Internate.'

Internegative. A negative coming out from a positive image.

Intertitles. A title card appearing intercut with a scene. This term is in contrast with subtitles. Intertitles are commonly used with silent films.

Iris. In cinephotography, an adjustable diaphragm of thin plates in front of a camera lens.

J

Jeopardy. Anything which engangers a character chances of attaining his story goal and fulfilling his desires.

Jidai-Geki films. Japan's popular period-films usually set in the Togukawa era (1616-1868). Jidai-Geki films like Kurosawas' Rashmon have been acknowledged and appreciated world-over.

Join. In editing, the splicing of two sections of film at a cut.

Joining the film pieces. Process of the pieces of the film to be joined are placed in the splicer with the teeth engaged in the sprocket holes and the emulsion side upwards. The two ends of the film are allowed to protrude beyond the hinged flaps. The emulsion from one piece is removed by means of a scraper. The flaps holding the second piece of the film is now closed. Thus trimming the protruding ends by a guillotine action. After brushing away any dust, the film cement is applied, with brush thinly and only on the scraped area. Immediately afterwards the splicer is closed this pressing the overlapping portion of the second piece of film into film contact with the first. Splice is placed under pressure from nearly twenty seconds to allow it to set. Thus the cement softens the base of both pieces of film and weld them together. During the process the film should not be hold by its surfaces but by its edges.

Judder. This term relates to the instability introduced when images sampled at one frame rate are converted to a different frame rate for viewing. This effect is most noticeable when frames are repeated or deleted in order to obtain slow motion or fast motion.

Jump cut. A cut involving in an interruption to the continuity of time. The effect is one of jerkiness and discontinuity. Jump cuts should always be avoided. Because of the jump cut the action in the first scene is not smoothly bridged to the action in the following scene and hence this cut is also called 'bad cut' in editing.

Juxtaposition. Telling a (film) story so that past and present, here and there, high and low, or any usually separate elements are in contact in the same story.

K

Kerr Cell. In sound recording, variable Density System is known as Kerr Cell. It is also called 'The Carolus Cell'. Kerr Cell is one of the fastest known means of modulating light, so there is no problem of getting adequate high-frequency response. However, the high voltage required, the discolouration of the liquid, geometrical limitations which restrict, the amount of transmitted light and most of all the nonlinearity of the characteristic, have contributed to the abandonment of the Kerr Cell as a sound recording device.

Key. A general adjective denoting importance like in key-factor.

Keyboard. In Music, a set of systematically arranged keys by which a machine is operated.

Key Grip. (Key Grip). The chief of a group of grips, often doubling for a construction co-ordinator and a back-up for the camera crew. Key grips closely work with the gaffer.

Key light. A shot's primary light source, which is primarily from one side.

Key line. Line of dialogue which reveals the heart of a story situation.

Key numbers. Numbers that are exposed on the film stock at regular intervals and that progress by one digit each time.

Kickoff. The start of production of principle photography.

Kinetoscope. A'talking machine' made by Edison whereby one person at a time could watch a 40 feet length of film passing through a series of rolls behind a powerful magnifying glass.

Kodachrome Process. Subtractive-type process wherein a superimposed layers of cyan, magnets and yellow dyes in the final film exert control of the primary colours viz. red, green, and blue. Kodachrome films if properly used give satisfactory colour rendering, but they are not intended for making precise colour records or for matching or measuring colours.

Kuleshov Effect. The effect obtained through juxtaposition in film editing. In the 1920s Russian Film Editor Lev Kuleshov (1899-1970) proved with his experiments that the human facial expression can be changed by altering the shots which they are intercut.

L

Lab. Dimunitive for Laboratory where the film is processed.

Lap Dissolve. Mixing up the end of two shots, end of one shot is to be mixed with the beginning next shot.

Lap Dissolve Sequence. (a) A series of time lapses (b) a series of transition and (c) a mixture of time lapses and transition.

Larry Edmunds Book Shop. World-known American bookshop which exclusive deals in film books/scripts etc. At times, shooting scripts on sale over here are in 2/3 drafts, which happens to be a useful source for comparative study of the scripts to the serious film-students.

Latent Image. The image made visible by developing the film which is formed on photographic emulsion by exposure to light.

Laterna Magica. A pertinent combination of film and live action very first successfully developed at the Brussels Exhibition (1958).

Lavendera (Lavender Print). Print in use between 1929 and 1940 replacing fine-grain print.

Lavialiere make. A small mocrophone pinned to the lapel or hanging about the neck of an actor.

Laying sound. To edit a sound track.

Layouts. (Blocking). A person responsible for working out the action before filming begins, included where the characters should be, and the camera angles.

Lazy-8. A special camera devised by Paramount in which the film magazinelie on their side and the film runs through the camera horizontally.

Lead Pole (Lead, Female Lead, Male Lead). The most important character in the movie, often distinguished by gender. This is basically a central character.

Leader. Extra film placed at the front or end of material which acts as protection to the body of a film.

Leadman. A team member of the art department, who is in charge of swing gangs and/or set dressers and reports to the set decorator.

Lecture-film. A film intended for use in academics, universities, research institutes and other centres of more advanced academic learning.

Legs. (Of a movie). Continuing to return large box-office figures.

Lens. A lens is a piece of transparent material (usually glass) bounded by curved surfaces which are generally spherical, including flat. Transparent substances have the property of bending, or refracting, rays of lights which fall obliquely, and the effect of the curvature of the surface is to cause all rays emanating from the point to be refracted so as to pass through a second point. The first is called the object point and the second is called the image point. Sir Christopher Wren was one of the first to make satisfactory lenses.

Lens, Anamorphic. The idea of an anamorphic image with a squeezed effect achieved as in a curved mirror was brought from China to Europe during the Renaissance. During these days painters made puzzle pictures by this means. Henry Chretien (1879-1956) devised this means for seeing a wide view out of the narrow aperture of the French military tank. He adapted the anamorphic lens for the still camera to make aerial photography more economical.

Lens Coating Process. In this process thin films of transparent material are applied to the optical surfaces of a lens system.

Letter boxing. (Letter box, Letter boxed). As the aspect ratio of movies are rarely the same as the aspect ratio of a television screen, when showing movies on television it is necessary to make sacrifices. Letter-boxing is the technique of shrinking the image just enough so that its entire width appears on the screen, with black areas above and below the image. There are both advantages and disadvantages of this technique, the advantage being the entire frame is always shown and the disadvantage is that the entire image must be shrink, which makes viewing on similar televisions more difficult. A term is in contrast with pan and scan.

Level Sync. The amount of volume heared (power or act of perceiving of sound) or electrically measured. Pitch at which the sound or picture records best.

Level. The relationship between separate picture and sound material i.e. sync-marked in parallel.

Library. (a) Collection of shots which may be useful for cutting into future films (b) Place where stock shots are stored and obtained.

Library Shot. A shot taken from a library or a film to use in a film.

License, Sync. Refer to Sync licence.

Light, the intensity of. The unity for the light intensity used to be the Hefner Candle (HK). Since 1948 a new unit has been adopted internationally and called the 'new candle' (NK). This name was later changed to 'Candela'

Lighting. (Lights). While filming for various technical and artistic reasons, most film-productions use artificial lighting. The lighting is used both on location or on a erected set. Lighting is designed by the Director of Photography mostly in consultation with the Director, and is the responsibility of the electrical department. Lit from various angles, actor, furniture, property and set can be induced to make the shot pictorially impressive. The sense of pattern is developed by the sharpness of high-light and shadow, or the sense of mystery deepened by the use of misty half-light produced by the device known as a soft focus or an image slightly blurred.

Lighting Crew. (Lighting technician, Lighting technicians). A group of technicians who instal, operate, and maintain lighting.

Lighting Department. The section of film production's responsible crew who attends to the job of lighting and other types of electrical works during filming.

Lighting, Front. See 'Front Lighting.'

Lighting Technician Characters. (LTCs). A member of the electrical department that is responsible for operating lights and lighting equipment on a set for the purpose of filming.

Lighting Valves. The first successful light valve for sound film recording was invented by Eugene Lauste.

Lighting (various) set-up. The placing of lights to illuminate a given shot or shots.

Lightness. The attribution of objects colours by which more or less of the incident light is reflected or lighted.

Limbo Shot. In effect a shot is stayed in space, with props, but without a normal set.

Line Producer. A producer who is responsible for meaning every person and issue during the making of a film.

Line Producers necessarily work on one film at a time since they have to give full justice to the film in hand.

Line of Sight. A straight line from an observer's eye to a distant point towards which he/she is looking.

Line, Tag. Please refer to Tag Line.

Lined Script. A copy of the shooting script which is prepared by the script supervision is called a Lined script. This script is mainly consisting of vertical line, line changing between straight and wavy and also of different lines. The main purpose of this script is to indicate during film-shooting (production) what coverage has had been shot till the day. A given vertical line indicates, via the line's start and end point what script material is covered in a particular shot, and whether given dialogue or action is on-screen or off-screen in the spot, indicated by the line changing between straight and wavy respectively. Different coloured lines usually represent certain type of shots like close-up, insert, steadicam, etc. Each vertical line is also notated with the slate of the shot e.g. "3C" etc. and a brief shot description e.g. "M2S Rolf & Liza". The lined script also frequently incorporates the script supervisor's script notes on the facing pages for a given scene.

The lined script is used by the film editor as a reference to what coverage was shot and to change made to the script during production. Lined scripts give editors an instant and a quick view of all the average coverage available, at a glance, so that he or she can make quick editing decisions without having to sort through all the footage repeatedly.

Lip Sync. Dialogue recorded in precise synchronization with the filming, so that speech and lip movements match the ability to duplicate the exact lip movement.

Live Area. (Safe Area) A camera's view-finder actually shows and records on film-stock a greater area of the scene then will appear in the final product. Makings are etched in the viewfinder to indicate to the camera operator the extents of the "viewable" film called the live area. An area beyond that (called the safe area) is also marked. It is in this area that the camera operator might direct the boom operator to place the boom microphone.

Live Action. Applied to the shooting of living things as opposed to abstract of animation filming.

Location Filming. (Location, On Location, Location Shooting) Filming which occurs at a place not constructed specifically for the purpose of film-production. Location filming is either outdoors, a well-known location or place which suffices for the purpose of shooting.

Location Manager. He is a responsible person of the film-unit who along with the assistance of his Assistant location manager manages various aspects of the film being shooted (filming) on location, such as previously arranging with the proper authorities for their permission to shoot in specific places.

Location Mixer. (In sound recording of films). A sound mixer responsible for mixing sounds recorded on location.

Location Scout. A person of the team of film production who looks for suitable locations for filming.

Lock it down. A direction given by the assistant director for everyone on the set to be quiet. It is called just prior to speed.

Lodz Film Schools. Polish Government set up this school in 1947 acknowledging the importance of cinema in Polish political and cultural life. World authority on film-education Jerzy Toeplitz was the first Principal of this school. During early 60s Toeplitz visited India. He had then given his expertise to the Film Institute of India in its formation days.

London International Film School. Having headquarters at 24 Shelton Street, London WC2 9HP this film-school conducts post-graduate Diploma in Film Production and Theory.

Long Focal Lens. Any lens of longer focal length than the normal standard focal length for the gauge of film in use.

Long Shot. (L.S) A shot that relates the subject to the background. Frequently it constitutes an orientation or establishing shot. A shot in which the camera is, appears to be, at a considerable distance from the subject. If the subject is the human figure, it would occupy about one third of the picture vertically.

Loop. In sound work, this usually means a continuous uninterrupted loop of track that makes a tone or sound effect for a mix. It is a continuous ribbon of film without beginning or end. Used for moving background in rear projection.

Loss of Light in Lenses. In passing through a lens, light is lost both by absorption and by reflection. The former loss is small, amounting to only some 2.4 per cent for each centimetre thickness of glass traversed.

Lot. Exterior set's erection is mostly done in the outside area of the studio. But in some cases in the open space of studio property this work is carried out. A term 'lot' denotes to this.

Low angle shot. A shot taken looking upward, is called a low angle shot.

Low Key. Under illumination of a scene to heighten dramatic action.

Low Key Lighting. Lighting in which dark, shadowy areas predominate as in most of horror films.

Lumiere Brothers. Auguste and Louis are the French inventors and pioneers of cinema. They arranged public performances of films at the selected countries. One of their representatives visited India and on July 7, 1896 he organised a film show at Esplanade Mansion (erstwhile Watson Hotel) in Mumbai then Bombay. Thereafter he continued to show these films for one full month.

Lyrics. The words sung in a (film) song. Musical compositions consisting of words written by poets/song writers.

M

Macguffin. (Weenie). The bone of contention in a film; the thing everyone is trying to save or steal. This term is used by Alfred Hitchcock to refer to an item, event or piece or knowledge that the characters in a film consider extremely important, but which the audience either doesn't know of or doesn't care about. Examples: the engine plans in 39 steps and the identity of the spy in North by Northwest.

Magazine. Light tight film-containers in which film is stored while used in a camera.

Magic Hour. Is the time which actually lasts 20 minutes or less when contrast is low and hues are most saturated, often with a rose cast. Film 'Days of Heaven, (1978) has been filmed almost entirely during magic hour.

Magnastripe. A magnetic tape using regular 35 mm perforated film base.

Magnetic Recording. Recording sound or pictures on plastic tape coated with iron oxide particles which are arranged or disarranged by magnetic action brought about electronically.

Magnetic Sound track. (Magnetic Print). A composite print in which the sound track is recorded on the attached strip of magnetic tape. Largely obsolete due to high cost and maintenance difficulties.

Magnetic Sound Film. Film that uses iron oxide as the coating on which sound is recorded and reproduced.

Maintenance Engineer. A person responsible for general maintenance and repair.

Majors. (In film industry). The major Hollywood Producer/ distributor studios (MGM/UA/20th Century Fox, Sony Pictures, Warner Brothers, Paramount Pictures, Universal and Disney).

Makeup. (Make up, Make-up Artist, Makeup Supervisor). The decorations placed directly on the skin or hair of an actor for cosmetic or artistic effect. Practitioners in this field are called artists or supervisors.

Maltese Cross. (Geneva Movement). Intermittent motion of the film is the basis of the motion picture, illusion. Stalwarts of Geneva Movement employed this mechanism in 35 mm projectors.

Married print. (Normal Print). Print of a sound film carrying both picture and sound track.

Martial-Arts. (Chop. sockey). A film which features hand to hand combat, usually using various Asian combat systems like Karate and the Chinese fighting styles popularly known in the west as Kung Fu. 'Chop socky' is a slang and scornful term for martial arts movies.

Martini Shot. Since the next shot' is in the Martini glass, the last shot of the working day/night is called a Martini shot. (See also Abby Singer shot).

Masc. A device used mostly in cameras and printers to limit the area of the frame that is exposed to light.

Masking. A term used to indicate the blocking out of part (usually the edges) of a photographic image.

Master Scene. An orientation shot (frequently a long one) taking in all or a considerable part of the action in an entire sequence.

Master Scene Script. A script (not the shooting script) which details the action and dialogue of a film.

Master Shot. A shot covering the action of a long scene but which is afterwards to be broken up by close-ups, cut-ins etc.

Matching. A term pertains to the continuity of the film. (Also applies to the process of cutting the negative).

Matte Artist. (Matte Paintings). A person who creates artwork (usually for the background of a shot) which is included in the movie either via a matter shot or optical printing.

Matte Shot. A photographic technique whereby artwork usually on glass — from a matte artist is combined with live action. A term is in contrast with back projection or a travelling matte.

Matte, Travelling. See 'Travelling Matte'—

MAVIKA. A digital camera for filming developed and launched by Sony.

Medic, Set. Refer the term 'Set, Medica.'

Medium Close-up. (MCU). A shot whose image size on the frame is between a medium shot and long shot.

Medium Long Shot. (MLS). A shot whose image size on the frame is between a medium shot and close-up.

Medium Shot. A shot of the subject in and of itself, with only incidental background.

Meter. (In music). Number of beats in a bar.

Method Acting. A style of acting formalized by Konstantin Stanislavsky (1863-1938) the Russian Stage Director. This typical style is known for character interpretation in acting. Stanislavasky's theory requires actors to draw experience from their own personal lives that correlate to the character they are playing—an extremely demanding process emotionally. In some cases, 'method' actors take the theory even further by arranging events in their private lives to resemble the lives of their characters.

Methods of Making films. See Film-making, Methods of.

Micky Mouse. Walt Disney's cartoon character which very first appeared as Mortimer Mouse' (1927) and eventually became very famous.

Miniature. A small-scale model of an object or set, used to cut the cost of filming airplane-crashes, floods, train wrecks etc.

Mini-microprocessor. A very small computer composed of one or more integrated circuits functioning as a unit.

Mini Majors. Studios which are large but not as large as the majors: Embassy, Gramercy etc.

Mini-Series. A television series with a set number of episodes which tell a complete story, usually filmed at the same time. In India for television serials minimum 13 episodes are considered. The term mini-series is in contrast with 'serial' which runs into several episodes.

Mise-en-scene. (Literally translated as "What's put into the scene", this is the sum total of all factors affecting the artistic 'look' or 'feel' of a shot or scene). These include shot selection/composition, production design and set decoration, as well as technical camera properties such as shutter speed, sperture, frame rate, and depth of field.

Missionary Statements. Of American/British University's Departments of Film-Courses: Now-a-days these Universities, as an expanding multi-cultural learning communities are running different courses relating to films and filming. Most of these Universities' mission statements declare that these Universities leading and broad-based universities serving national, regional and institutional needs and characterized by quality and provision, access to flexible and relevant higher film/ TV/Video education and the development of the full human potential of film students.

Mix. Applied to sound. This describes the process of combining two or more sound sources into a single recording. Mix (Noun) is resultant sound track with regard to picture. See Dissolve (Lap Dissolve).

Mockumentary. Hybrid form of films which both evokes realism and pokes fun at it. Mockumentary implies a particular structure for the story-the rise and fall of a film or television show, a weekly episode of television and also the day-long production of a soap opera.

Modulate. To vary the amplitude, frequency of phase of the carrier wave or signal by combining with a wave of a different frequency, so as to transmit a radio, television, etc. signal.

Modules in Film & Television Studies. Considering the fact that arts and humanities courses develop some of the most useful skills employees values value. Faculty of Arts of Brune University, Uxbridge UB8 3PH(UK) is offering a varied curriculum too its students in its Film and television studies. Most of the other Universities are also offering their subjects on the same lines.

The following modules in three different levels is available at the Brunel University, U.K.

Level 1: Introduction to Film and Television, Audio Visual Theory and Practice, Critical Methodologies, The Development of the Moving Image, A Case of Study British Film and TV in the 1960s.

Level 2: Video Production, TV; Forms & Meanings; Science Fictions, New Hollywood Cinema, Photography: Theory & Practice (Single honours students only), European Cinema, British Film & Television, Melodrama: A Thematic Study, Hong Kong Cinema.

Level 3: Documentary; Theory & Practice, Special Project (Dissertation), Activism and Television, Gender and Sexuality, Third Cinema, Psycho-analysis and the Moving Image. The Horror Film, Comedy, Death and the Moving Image.

Maureen Moren, Dean, Faculty of Arts of Brunel University has had mentioned in it's booklet that, "...Our aim is to provide you with the necessary analytical and research skills with which to investigate the subject area in terms of culture, history, context, the politics of representation, and aesthetics. The video production work undertaken on the programme is designed to provide you with the opportunity to experience some of the choices that have to be made in the creation of audio visuals. At the core of all our modules is the close analysis of film and television texts, which will included the analysis of your own creative work in the practical modules. Throughout the programme you will be able to explore your own ideas and interests in relation of audio-visual texts and critical theory. While on Brunel's Film and Television studies degree course you will see a diverse range of texts from Hollywood to African Cinema, Godard to Carry on, The Piano to the Terminator; On the Buses to Ad Fab and from Panorama to South Park..."

Montage. An artistic device for creating an artistic 'look' or 'feel' of a scene, through the use of visual editing. Often in contrast with mise-en-scene. This term was originally used to describe creative editing by the Russians in the 1920s.

Mood Music. Music used to compliment or support the atmosphere and emotional content of a scene which is dramatic, gay, sad, pastoral etc.

MOS. (Mit-out-Sound). A gag line referring to shots or sequences to filmed silent.

Moscow Film Festival. The First International Film Festival in Eastern Europe held in Moscow (1935).

Motion Artifact. (Nyquist Limit, Strobing). The visual interference patterns between a shot's frame rate and a film object's periodic motion or change. If a film shot is filmed with a frame rate R, any images of periodic events of a frequency greater than R/2 (the Nyquist limit) will be misrepresented of film. A commonly-occurring example of this artifact is the illusion of spoked wheels appearing to turn in the wrong direction or at the wrong rate.

Motion Blur. Shots of objects that quickly move in the camera's frame and/or shots with a slow shutter speed are likely to produce a 'smearing' effect, since the object is in the range of positions during a single exposure.

Motion Capture. An animation technique in which the actions of an animated object are derived automatically from the motion of a real world actor or object.

Motion Control. A camera set up which records the motion of a camera during a shot so that visual effects can be easily synchronized with the scene photographed.

Motion Picture. Also called movie, film, flick and picture.

Motion Picture Association. (Also Motion Picture Export Association of America. (MPEAA). The Motion Picture Association of America (MPA) and its international counterpart. The Motion Picture Association serve as the voice and advocate of the American motion picture, home video and television industries, domestically through the MPAA and internationally through the MPA. Before 1994, the MPA was known as the Motion Picture Export Association of America.

Motion Picture Association of America. (MPAA). This organization founded in 1921, through the classifications and Ratings Administration (CARA) issues certificates.

Motion Picture Parent Company. (MPCC). An American Trust founded in January 1909 for parents.

Motion Picture Producers & Distributors of America. (MPPDA). Official organization established by American film producers and distributors.

Motion Picture Production. Main steps to be taken for—

Ordinarily for the production of motion picture the main steps will have to be taken in different fields. Of all these the following aspects are very important:

(A) Blue Print. Getting the facts, contract, story out-line, shooting script (B) Preliminaries: Casting, choosing locations, building sets properties and costumes. (C) Art Work: Art for titles, shooting title, art for animation sound, shooting animation. (D) Shooting; direction, camera, sync, production stills (E) Editing: selecting scenes, work printing, editing, master cutting (F) Recording; Musical score,.sound effects, narration, final recording. (G) Laboratory: Special effects, timing original, first print, release prints, & (H) Distribution.

Motivation. The logical basis for a character's action.

Moving Short. (Travel Shot). A shot made from the moving vehicle.

Moviola. A sound/picture viewing device used in film-editing.

Multimedia. Software that uses sound, video, text, graphics and so on in combination to provide news ways of presenting into and interacting with it.

Multiplane Camera. In animated films Walt Disney Studio devised this rostrum to produce realist effects of depth and perspectives.

Multiplex. A theatre with multiple screening grooms/halls/ auditoriums, allowing it to show several films at one time. In early August 2001 Government of Maharashtra announced special monetary concessions for establishing 'multiplex' in its state.

Music Editor. A person who prepares printed parts from the composer's score for the musicians to play from at the score recording sessions.

Music Supervisor. Musical Director, Musical Direction, Music Director, Music Direction)

A person who co-ordinates the work of the composer, the editor and sound mixers.

Musical film. A movie whose dramatic story structure includes unrealistic episodes of musical performance and/or dancing.

Mute. A shot without sound.

N

Nagra. A quarter-inch tape recorder.

Narration. Words spoken over the film either by anonymous person or by a person or actor who figures in the film.

National Film Archive. London. This archive was established in 1935 as the National Film Library under Ernest Lindgren. In 1961, the Articles of Association of the British Film Institute—the Archive's parent body—were extended to include television, and the Archive began to select and acquire television material for preservation.

National Film Archive of India. (NFAI). This organisation established by the Ministry of Information and Broadcasting of Government of India in Pune (Maharashtra) and is engaged in the task of preservation of the important Indian films for prosperity. The Archives has in its Library films from many countries of the world, besides India. NFAI launched in February 1964 joined the International Federation of Film Archives at early stages which enabled NFAI to establish in the beginning rapport with 40 Archives in different countries in the world. Film Institute of India's Principal Jagat Murari, Prof. Satish Bahadur and film-historian B.V. Dharap were instrumental in giving the present status to NFAC.

National Film Board of Canada was set up in May 1939 as a result of a report by John Crierson (1898-1972) (who first applied the word 'documentary' to cinema. Later he became this Board's first Chairman.

National Film Theatre. A club cinema established and run by the British Film Institute. This located in London (England).

NC-17 of MPAA. (No one of the age 17 & under admitted). NC-17 is also known as X-Rated. A certificate issued by the MPAA indicating that no person aged 17 or under will be allowed to attend a screening of the movie. This MPAA's category was formerly called 'X', but many filmgoer's mistaken association of 'X' films with XXX films caused the MPAA to change this on September 27, 1990.

Negative. Original film exposed in the camera from which positive prints can be made.

Negative Cost. The cost of a movie through the production of a finished negative. The cost towards the prints, advertising or distribution is not included in the negative cost.

Negative Cutter. A person of the team who matches the negative of a movie and conforms (matches) it to the final version of the film as decided by the film-makers. From this negative only the prints are made.

Negative Pick-up. An agreement where a distribution acquires a finished negative and agrees to pay P&A and distribution costs. This is as opposed to deals where the distribution is involved during production.

Negative Print. (Negative, Neg.) The film-print that is having dark for light and light for dark used in the camera.

N.G. SHOTS/TAKES. Shots/takes that are no good and therefore not worth using in the cutting while film editing.

Neo-realism. A term first applied by the critic Pietrangeli which gives accent on Italian Cinema's Verism (use of everyday contemporary material) style.

Neon lighting ad. Sir W.M. Ramsay (1852-1916) founded a gas in the atmosphere which gave an advantage to the advertising agencies to give a red glow for ad-signs. Thanks to Ramsay, neon lighting is being used by the film industry in various colours.

Newsreel. First produced by Lumiere Brothers, for the purpose of demonstrations of their equipment etc.

Newsreels (In India). After taking over the Indian Movietone News Government of India in September 1943 renamed it 'The Indian News Parade. Afterwards the newsreels came to be produced every week in English and also in addition to the four Indian regional languages.

Night Films. This category, like 'Spy' films has been formed from its very nature. Kobita Sarkar who had been a Member of the Advisory Penal of the Central Board of Film Censors in Mumbai (then Bombay) and Calcutta from 1964 to 1977—except for two short breaks, in one of which she was Member of the Board writes about 'Night Films' as follows, "Night Films were on the whole like a series of filmed cabaret shows, without much aesthetic appeal, were possible entertainment'. These were rarely vulgar in the broader sense of the term, though inevitably there was a degree of undress.... The corrupting influence of the cinema on their youth and accusing it of not sufficiently cautious about things in the night films. Often their titles were more suggestive and risque than the contents... (from 'You can't please Everyone').

Nitrate Film. Until 1951, Nitrate film was being used for 35mm though fire risks were there while filming. Thereafter less flammable material used negative film came into practice.

Noise Reduction. Dolby. See Dolby, Noise Reduction.

Non-linear Editing. The computer-assisted editing of a movie without the need to assemble it in linear sequence. This term is 'the visual equivalent of word-processing.

Non-theatrical Film. Ordinarily, a film shown in churches, clubs, schools, and colleges etc. which are used to inform, influence and inspire, rather than to entertain.

Notch. Shallow cuts on edges of a film to warn laboratory technicians of timing changes to be made in a printer.

Number Board. Board photographer at the beginning of takes carrying shot number. This team is also names as claper-board and slate.

Nut. Operating expenses to be recovered, often deductible in an exhibitor's contract with distributors.

Nutral Density Filters. Filters that reduce the amount of light entering the camera.

Nychthemeron Shooting. This term refers to the film shooting scheduled for day-night. (i.e. 24 hours) shooting wherein the artists/technicians work in shifts but the shooting work is in progress.

Nykvist's Lighting Technique. This term is named after Sevn Nykvista Swedish cameraman who while working with Bergman has had mastered this lighting technique. For Bergman's and later for this own films Nykvist based on his own experiments with coated stock and by a control observation of landscape had used this technique with great skill.

O

Oater. Western film.

Oberhausen Film Festival was started in 1955 by Helmar Hoffman who had determined when a prisoner-of-war in Scotland to launch a project to bring nations together in friendship. Oberhousen quickly became the most distinguished festival in Europe for short films.

Obligatory Scene. A film's climatic confrontation, the elements for which have been planned.

Off-beam. Speaking into a microphone outside the angle of pick-up.

Offbeat film. A film produced out of the usual conventional style.

Off-camera. Beyond the margin of the film-frame.

Off-screen. (Also on screen space). Areas defined by the limits of the film-frame.

O.K. Takes. Shots which are good enough to be printed.

One-one. (1-1). An exact copy of the dialogue track as composed by the film editor.

Open (Opens, Opened, Opening) This term refers to the time at which a movie is first released in the theatres. Movies will very often open at different times in different countries/regions.

Opening Weekend. When a movie is first released in each country, its success is often measured in terms of its gross for the first weekend it opened. A disproportionate number of people usually see a movie on its opening weekend and therefore box-office numbers are a good guide as to whether the movie will be a hit or not.

Opportunity Forecast of the film. This is a form of business forecast in film trade in which an effort is made to predict future conditions in the marketplace which might present opportunities for exhibiting new and brand films in the theatres. In India for example before the so called 'fixing' problems ordinarily new films were not released for the first time during the days of Test Cricket Matches. Similarly, film-distributors in India manage to continue or exhibit his new film during the Deepawali Light Festivals.

Optical Effects. (Opticals). The penumbra of effects obtainable by use of the optical printer at the laboratory.

Optical Printer. (Optical Printing). A laboratory machine for combining the image of one or more reels of film through photographic techniques. This is in contrast with digital compositing.

Optical Soundtrack. A composite print in which the soundtrack is recorded via the varying width of a transparent track which runs beside the sequence of frames on a print.

Opticals. Fades, mixes, wipes, superimposition added during the process of printing a film.

Orchestral Arrangements. (Arrangements, Orchestrations, Orchestration). An adaptation of the score for all instruments in an orchestra. (See also arranger.)

Orchestrator. A person who writes orchestral arrangements.

Ordinance, Cable, Television. (Indian). Indian cable/ television ordinance was first promulgated on

September 29, 1994. In January, 1995, the President Dr. S.D. Sharma repromulgated it. Under this Ordinance, all the cable operators in India were required to register themselves. In accordance with the regulation it was essential to transmit two doordarshan (Indian T.V. Centres satellite channels and in case of replacement of equipments they should meet the criteria formulated by the Bureau of Indian Standards. This Ordinance tries to channelise the cable TV operations in the country and limits foreign equity in such networks to 49 per cent. The Ordinance empowers the Central Government of India to seize and confiscate the equipment of cable operators who break the rules and punish them by finding as well as imprisoning the defaulters. The Government can prohibit the transmission of programmes which are not in public interest. During September 2000 representatives of the Indian Cable Union had prolonged discussions with the Hon. Minister of Information & Broadcasting regarding modifying certain rules in the Ordinance. A new reformist attitude towards certain rules and regulations is being taken in this context.

Organisation Catholique Internationale du Cinema et de l'Audiovisuel'. (OCIC). International Catholic Organization for Cinema and Audiovisual. Since, 1935, this organization has been officially recognised as the official organization of the Catholic Church in the field of cinema.

Original. (In editing). The material on which the image have been photographed.

Orthochromatic Emulsions. The term applies to emulsions whether on plates or films, that have been rendered sensitive to green and yellow light. Although sensitised to yellow and green, will show that the orthochromatic plate or film shall remains a disproportionately high sensitivity to value.

Orthohcromatic film. The black and white film that is not read sensitive is called the orthochromatic film.

Oscar Academy Award. Coveted prize in the form of a gold statuette awarded annually by the American Academy of Motion Picture Arts & Sciences. The statuette was executed by George Stanley from rough sketches made by Cedric Gibbons. Many a people believe that this award is name after Oscar Wilde—talented 19th century playwright, but it's not true. As the anecdote goes, during the initial stages when this statue was being prepared, Margaret Herrick, then Librarian at AMPAS and later its Executive Director exclaimed that 'OH! He looks like my uncle OSCAR'. The same name was thereafter retained. The award is restricted to American films, but there is an annual award for the best foreign film. In 1992, Special Oscar Award of Akademi of Motion Pictures, Hollywood was announced for Satyajit Ray. During this period Ray was stuck in the hospital after his severe heart ailment. Hollywood's special team of cinematographers and senior officials therefore specially came down to Calcutta to cover this special event. Unfortunately after few months this celebrated event took place in America and Ray was given OSCAR posthumously, by presenting on the screen the film taken in the hospital. (See also 'Winners' of Oscar Awards')

Out of Sync. When the performer's lip movements are not synchronized with sound on track. It can result from bad editing or incorrect threading in projector.

Out-Take. (Out take, Outtake/s). A take of a scene not used in a movie. In some movies, out takes are shown under the closing credits.

Overcranking. The process of speeding the frame rate of a camera up, so that when the captured pictures are played at the normal up, so that when the captured pictures are played at the normal frame rate the action appears to be in slow motion. Historically, cameras were operated by turning a crank at a constant required speed; hence, 'overcranking' refers to turning the crank too quickly.

Overlapping Dialogue. The overlap of the speed of the character with that of another.

Oxford Companion to Film, ed. by Liz-Anne Bawden, Lecturer in Film, Slade School of Fine Art, University College, London and published by Oxford University Press is being recognized as the 'Bible's on the Films and Film-making.

Ozoner. A slang for a drive-in theatre.

Ozu's Indoor Sequences. In the indoor sequence Yasujiro Ozu (1903-63) is considered to be the highly respectable because of his indoor sequences which he use to prefer in almost all his films. These were always shot from a very low camera angle, approximately to the eye level of people sitting on the floor.

P

P&A Costs. Prints and advertising are the major costs of film distribution.

Pace. The rate of delivery.

Packaged Environment. A physical entity such as a theme park, stadium, shopping mall or cultural centre which has a highly developed identity calculated to enhance the presentation of products/goods and services. Entertainment complexes such as Disney World are the most elaborate packaged environments.

Painter. Stand by. Please see 'Stand by Painter'.

PAL. A standard for television/video display popular in Europe and Australia. The standard for TV/video display in the United States and Canada is called NTSC.

Pan. The action of rotating a camera about its vertical axis. Also used for the movement between the two characters not contained within the camera frame. (Pan is the abbreviation of Panorama).

Pan blur. Quick pan which blurs the scene beyond recognization.

Pan and Scan. (Panned and Scanned). The technique of chopping off strips from one or both sides of the picture when displaying. The areas chopped off are typically changed on a shot-by-shot basis, depending on scene composition. The main advantage of this technique is that it allows detail to be seen, the disadvantage is that shot composition is sometimes destroyed.

Parallax. Due to the lens and view-finder being in different positions, the difference between the image seen throughout the view-finder and the image recorded by the lens vary. Parallax is the difference between these two components.

PG. (Parental Guidance Suggested). A certificate issued by the MPAA indicating that a film's content is suitable for viewing by children but recommends parental guidance.

Paravision. 3-D system developed at Paramount Studios.

Peripheral Vision. Side vision of the amount one sees on each side, when looking straight ahead.

Persistence of vision. The retention of an image of a viewed subject on the retina of the viewer for the fraction of a second after the subject has been removed.

PG-13. A certificate introduced by the MPAA on July 1, 1984 to indicate that a movie's content is rated a slightly stronger than a PG certificate.

Perma-mix. One of the end products of the mix process.

Pete Smith. Specialities. One of the best known of the numerous series of short films (fillers) issued by Hollywood studios.

Photography, Additional. See Additional Photography.

Photography, Time Lapse. See Time Lapse Photography.

Photomacrography. Photography with image magnifications greater than the actual size.

Pickups. (Picked up). 1. Movies made by one studio that have been acquired by another, 2. Any recording OR pictorial shots needed to correct the original, 3.

A microphone or a television camera for converting sound or an image into electrical signals.

Picture Car. A vehicle shown in a movie.

Picture work. See work picture.

Pipeline. A schedule of movie projects in production.

Pixelation. A variant of stop-motion animation where actors are the objects being filmed. The key example is 'Neighbours produced in 1952.

Plant. Establishment of an idea, character and property to be used more significantly later in the film. For example, a gun is seen in a drawer when the same is opened to get a pad or pencil.

Play-back. (In sound recording). The playing of previously recorded, both for reference or simply to check its quality.

Plot. A writer's dramatized plan of action for manipulating emotions of audience. A plot is the entanglement of incidents. Plot is not to be confused with a story or a situation. Polt has stated that there are only 36 plots (basic) and that all the stories are basically permutations or/and combinations of these plots. They are as follows:

1. Supplication, 2. Deliverance, 3. Crime followed by vengeance, 4. Vengeance, kindred upon kindred. 5. Pursuit, 6 Disaster, 7. Falling prey to cruelty of misfortune, 8. Revolt, 9. Daring enterprise, 10. Abduction, 11. The Enigma, 12. Obtaining, 13. Enmity of Kinsman, 14. Rivalry of kinsman, 15. Murderous adultery, 16. Madness, 17. Fatal Imprudence, 18. Involuntary Crimes of Love, 19. Slaying of a Kinsman unrecognised, 20. Sacrificing self for an ideal, 21. Self sacrifice for kindred, 22. All sacrificing for a passion, 23. Necessity of sacrificing loved ones, 24. Rivalry of superiors and Inferiors, 25. Seduction, 26. Obstacles to love, 27. Discovery of the dishonoured of a loved one, 28. Crimes of love, 29. An enemy loved, 30. Ambition,

31. Mistaken jealousy, 32. Erroneous judgement, 33. Remorse, 34. Recovery of a lost one, 35. Loss of loved ones, 36. Conflict with God.

Point of View. (PoV). A camera angle in which the camera views what would be visible from a particular object's position. The abbreviation is often used in a slug line.

Pornographic film. (Porno, Skin, Flick). A film in which sex is graphically depicted to a large degree.

Positive Print. Print from a negative. This is a normal print suitable for projection.

Post-Production. (Postproduction, post). Work performed on a movie after the end of principal photography. Usually involves editing and visual effects.

Post-Production Co-ordinating. A production assistant working for the post-production supervisor.

Post-Production Supervisor. A person of the team directly reporting to the Producer of the film. He works side by side with the Director of the film as well as with the Editor of the film. His main responsibility rests with the task of satisfying the wants of the Director in respect of the film being shooted and to finish the film in given time and budget. Post-production Supervisor's typical duties include of controlling all activitics with vendors such as optical houses, sound facilities, inserts, re-shooting, score, delivery requirements to domestic and international distributors, legal clearances, colour timing, preview screening, video mastering etc.

Post-synchronization. Recording sound to a picture after the picture has been shot.

Predicament. A situation emotionally disturbing tc the central character is a screenplay that he is impelled to take action directed at the changing said situation.

Pre-production. (Preproduction, Pre). Arrangements made before the start of the actual filming. This can include script editing, set construction, location scouting and casting.

Premiere. (Bow, Debute). The first official public screening of a movie, marking the opening. Premiere event is often a gala event attended by the film-makers, stars and other celebrities.

Premise. A hypothetical 'What if-?' question that provides the basic idea for and springboard to a film story.

Prequal. A movie that presents the characters and/or events chronologically before the setting of a previously filmed movie.

Presentation, Feature. See Feature Presentation.

Presenter —(Presents.) A presenter is a person-often or well respected—who introduces a movie or show on screen on voice—over. Some films include a credit 'presented by' or 'Presents', which indicates that the person is an executive producer as opposed to someone who appears in the film.

Preview, Sneak. See Sneak Preview.

Principal Photography. (Principal Filming, Principal, Shoot) The filming of major or significant of a movie which involve lead actors.

Print. A projectionable version of a movie, usually consisting of one or more reels. When referring to a particular take on a continuity report, 'print' indicates that the take should be developed.

Print, Answer. See 'Answer Print'.

Print, Commage. BBC coined this term which refers to a print with picture and magnetic sound combined on the same piece of film.

Print, Comopt. A print with picture and optical sound combined on the same piece of film.

Print, Composite. See Composite Print.

Print, Positive. See Positive Print.

Printer, Light. The source of illumination in a printer.

Printing. Exposed picture negative and exposed sound negative should be printed keeping the distance of nearly 19½ frames, to suit the arrangement of the picture light and sound light in the projector. This is done in the laboratory. In the case of 16 mm film, however, the difference is of 26 frames.

Printing, Contact. *See* Contact Printing.

Printing Machines. The production of printing machines may be divided into six groups:

(i) Intermittent, or step by step, contact printers.

(ii) Intermittent, or step by step, optical printers.

(iii) Continuous rotary optical printers.

(iv) Continuous optical printers.

(v) Continuous rotary contact printers to printers, and

(vi) Continuous rotary contact printers to print both picture and sound.

Process Shot. A shot in which foreground action is staged against a translucent screen on which a filmed background is projected.

Processing Tanks. The processing tanks consist of 5 water-tight compartments comprising (i) The developing tank which is nearest the splicing table and has a capacity of 36 gallons and holds 6 film racks, (ii) The 2 fixing tanks 13½ gallons each and hold 2 film racks. The developing and fixing tanks each contain a coiled stainless tube (steel) used to circulate heating or cooling water through the tanks. The circulating pump is connected with the developing tank and to avoid possible corrosion, is fitted with a wrought iron rotor and a monel-metal spindle. A series of valves are fitted between the pumps and the processing tanks to enable pump to be used for different purposes.

Producer. (Prod). The chief of a movie production in all matters save the creative efforts of the director.

Product Placement. A business arrangement whereby the film-makers agree to show the products or logo of a particular company, usually in return for payment or other consideration.

Production Accountant. (Accountant). The person responsible for managing finances during the production.

Production Assistant. (PA). (Gopher, Set Production Assistant). A person responsible for various jobs, such as stopping traffic, acting as couriers, fetching items from craft service. These PAs are often attached to individual actors or filmmakers.

Production Buyer. A person who purchases supplies, equipment and property necessary for a film-production.

Production Company. A general term for a company that is associated with the making of a movie.

Production Date. (Production). In the film industry this term refers to the phase of movie making during which principal photography occurs. Popularly, however, 'production' means the entire movie project.

Production Designer. (Production Design). An artist responsible for designing the overall visual appearance of a film.

Production Illustrator. (Storyboard Artist, Illustrator). A person from the team responsible for drawing the storyboards and anything else that needs to be drawn during the production of the films.

Production Manager. (PM). Production Co-ordinator/ Supervisor) Reporting to the film's producer, this person is responsible for all the practical matters such as ordering equipment, getting near-location, accommodation for the cast and crew set.

Production Report. A daily report of actual progress versus the production schedule. He has also to register explanations of unexpected events.

Production Report. A copy of sound recorded for a given scene.

Production Schedule. A detailed plan of the timing at the activities associated with the making of a film, of particular interest to production managers.

Production Secretary. He is a Secretary to Production Manager.

Production Sound Mixer. The Head of the Sound Recording Department of the set. He is responsible for the process of recording all sync dialogue and sync sound effects in a scene.

Progression. Forward movement of a screenplay towards the climax through incorporation of new information and development.

Projectionist. A studio/cinema employee that operates a projector.

Projector. A device for displaying a reel of a film on screen, either for the screening or a back projection.

Projector. Double Head. See Double Head Projector.

Promotion Marketing Association of America. (PMAA). A New York based Association of promotion service companies, sales incentive organizations and related businesses. PMAA's membership also includes manufacturers of premium merchandise, consultations and advertising agencies as associated members. The association studies and promotes premium usage and co-sponsors both the New York Premium Show and the National Premium Show. Many-a film and Video ad agencies have shown their interest in becoming associated members of the PMAA.

Prop. An object on the set used by an actor e.g. phones, guns, cutlery etc.

Property Assistant. (Prop. Assistant). A person in the team responsible for the maintenance of props on a set.

Property Master. (Prop. Master, Props, Property, Asst. Prof. Master). A person in a team responsible for buying/acquiring any props needed for film-production. This term is in contrast with set dresses. Property Master is generally in contact with rental houses or is responsible for purchasing and handling props and picture-vehicles.

Proportioning. The matching of emphasis to importance in a film-script.

Proposal Outline. A brief statement of purpose, target audience, concept and specifications for a proposed fact film.

Prosthetic Appliances. (Prosthetic Make-up, Prosthetic). Make up that requires gluing additions (prosthetic appliances) made of a material such as latex or gelatin in an actor's skin. This may be applied by someone other than the designer. See also 'Squib.'

Protagonist. A film's main character.

Protection shot. An admission of failure or insecurity.

Publicity Assistant. Assistant to the Publicity Director. Besides the jobs assigned by the Publicity Director. P.A. prepares write-ups, material for the print or electronic media (usually in the form of exclusive/latest news/interviews) which may stimulate the interest of the film-goers or enhance the reputation of a person in the film in hand.

Publicity Department. (Advertising). The section of a production's crew responsible for promoting a movie. Individual positions within in this department include: Publicity Director, Publicity Assistant and Still Photographer.

Publicity Director. (Unit Publicist). Chief of the publicity department responsible for promoting the media's publicity.

Puffery. (artistic license). A slightly exaggerated advertisement or publicity made of film under production/ready for release.

Pull-Back. A shot which re-establishes a scene after a series of close shots.

Pull Strategy. (Sometimes also known as pull-through marketing). A marketing distribution strategy in which a film's promotional efforts are directed in an effort to create strong theatre-owners' demand for a new film being released.

Pulsing. In film-advertising, pulsing is a strategy designed to build filmgoers awareness. Marketers of the film-distribution system using this strategy expend advertising money and effort in periodic spurts or waves.

Pulsation. In music, this means the alternating 6—cycle current being recorded on one channel of a magnetic tape.

Punch. Hole in film or flash effect on video tape.

Pure Monopoly. A film-oriented market condition in which there is a single seller of a film or flash effect on video tape.

Purpose of Films. (i) Entertainment (ii) Information (iii) Propaganda, (iv) Historical Record, (v) Education & (vi) Monetary benefits.

Pyrocatechol. A phenol made synthetically for using especially as a photographic developer.

Q

'Q' Certificate. In India, in March 1979 'Q' certificate for films was mooted. This is aimed at the direction of quality and is to be given to the Indian films which do not contain 'crudity and other objectionable or adverse characteristics'. A film-maker who gets this 'Q' certificate is entitled for getting exemption from various taxes.

Quality of a Print refers to a degree of excellence or fineness.

Quarter. A quarter of the year; 3 months. For financial issues film-production accounts and publicity departments use this term.

Quarter-inch Tape. The usual vehicle for original sound recording when filming.

Quartz Lighting. A common but technically incorrect term used to describe tungsten halogen lamps.

Quartz (qualified) Crystal. A crystal; used in cameras and recorders.

Quick-five Cameras. Equipped with special mechanism for winding on the film and resetting the shutter.

Quick Save. A resolution of a film's problem in less time than it seems believable.

Quid. A slang for a pound sterling in U.K.

Quota. National Government's move to support their own film industry by specifying the proposition of their films to be exhibited to important films.

Quota Quickies. (Low Budget). This term refers to the films having short subjects made in the United Kingdom in 1930s. The Cinematographic Films Bill, passed in April 1927 stipulated that all the U.K. cinemas will have to include a proportion of British films in their programmes. The percentage varied rising to 20 per cent at one time. The 'Quota Quickies" were generally of a quite low quality but there also some gems hidden in their midst, notably those by Michael Powell of 'Rynox' (1931).

R

'R' (Restricted). A certificate issued by the MPAA indicating that persons under the age of 16 would only be admitted when accompanied by an adult. The age was later raised to under 17 years old and varies in some jurisdictions.

Rack-over. In filming up a scene the lens or camera mechanism is made moved aside to enable the cameraman to see the scene as it will be taken through the lenses and from this to adjust his view finder.

Rain, Creating of. Many art directors prefer building vast grids of 2" iron barrel that zig-zag tne set and that have 5 perforations 1" apart on the top. A house pipe is harnessed to either end of the zig-zag more or less pressure is added according to the extent to which the coks are opened.

Rate, Frame Rating. See Frame Rating Rate.

RAY (S.) FILM & TELEVISION INSTITUTE. The Institute has been named after Satyajit Ray, the celebrated Indian Film Director. This Institute is located at Calcutta. The Oxford Companion to Film edited by Liz-Anne Bawden remarks, '...Rays films express an appealing humanism as well as an engaging love of cinema; and he has evolved a personal style in which an assured yet sensitive synthesis of eastern and western values assures him an audience in both countries..' See also Satyajit Ray Film & T.V. Inst.

Reader. An employee of a studio's scenario department whose job is to read, synopsize and at times pass judgement on literacy and dramatic properties for the purpose of motion picture production.

Reaction Shot. A short or part of a short that is taken or used to show the reaction of one or more characters to action and/or sound that proceed it.

Release Print. Projection print of a finished print is called a release print.

Reproductions. (In music) The photo-copying of the musical score.

Re-recording Mixer. In sound recording, a Member of the sound crew responsible for mixing the final sound elements (dialogues, music, sound effects and foley). In most feature films and some of the television shows there is crew of 3 re-recording mixers one for dialogue, one for sound effects and foley and one for music). Sometimes in the television, the music mixer mixes the foley for expediency. There are also 2-person crew in which the dialogue mixer (generally considered the lead mixer) mixes music as well, with the other person mixing sound effects and foley.

Rear Projection. Projection of a film onto a translucent screen from behind, in order to provide background for live foreground action.

Reel. A strip of film wound on a metal wheel. The typical reels hold 15 to 25 minutes of film.

Release Print. A finished sound print for projection. When a movie is shipped to exhibitors by distributor, it is deemed to have been released for public viewing— there are no longer any studio restrictions on who can see the movie.

Relief. A sequence or sequences designed to reduce audience tension, often through humour, after a period of high excitement.

Resolution. The defeat of desire by danger or vice-versa in consequence of the protagonists behaviour in the ultimate conflict that is the climax.

Re-take. (Re-take). Repetition of a film shot (take).

Reverberation time. The time taken for a sound on its cessation or a pause at its source, to die away the inaudibility.

Reversal film. A typical filmstock which after exposure and processing produces a positive image instead of a negative without an intermediary process.

Reverse angle. A view i.e. 180 degree from the preceding shot.

Rising Action. Also Complications. Events that build the dramatic interest until a climax is reached.

Rock & Roll Recorder. A studio recorded and sound mixing equipment that can be reversed to enable corrections of wrongly recorded sounds to be recorded immediately.

Roll. Any section of a film that is wound on itself or core (bobbin) or on a spool.

Room Tone. Different sets and locations have different audio characters. A sound recordist will typically make a recording of the natural ambient 'silence' in a set/ location for the sound editor, who will use it as a reference point, or for when silence is required.

Rotoscoping. (Rotoscope). An animation technique in which images of live action are traced. These images are traced wither manually or automatically. She also motion capture.

Rough cut. First and over length assembly of shots into a work print arranged into their proper sequences.

Rube Goldberg Device. Any ridiculously over complex machine designed to perform a simple basic talk.

Running Gas. The building up of the humour of some incident or fragment of behaviour by repetition as a film progresses.

Rushes. The unedited picture and sound material of any shoot. First prints of scenes usually projected daily for approval of various authorities.

—

S

Saccade Frame. A jerky frame in the shots. This rapid movement jumps from fixation on one point to another.

Safe Area. Basically a camera's viewfinder actually shows and records on film stock a greater area of the scene than will appear in the final product. Marking are etched in the viewfinder to indicate to the camera operator the extents of the viewable film which is called the live area. An area beyond that is called the safe area. It is in this safe area that the production sound mixer might direct the boom operator to place the boom microphone. Also see Live Area.

Sahani, Balraj. National Award. This coveted award is instituted by a Shimla-based All India Artists' Association and is presented to the most popular Hindi Film of the year.

Sampling. (In sound recording). The recording of a sound effect, or a note from the musical instrument. This enables to vary length or pitch of the sound.

Satyajit Ray Film & Television Institute. This institute is functioning as a premier training institute in Bengal, India. It is located at E.M. Bye Road, Calcutta 700 094. See also 'Ray Film & T.V. Institute.

Scenario. The story of the film in its final form, from which the Director works during production. It usually contains a detail description of the action shot, together with settings and camera position.

Scenario Writing Problems in. (i) Deciding the structure for the film-story, (ii) Treating the film-story for sound and for action, (iii) Making use of camera, (iv) Proper use of dialogue, (v) Possibilities of tempo and rhythm and (vi) Avoiding common faults.

Scene. A piece of action which appears to be continuous on the screen though it may be composed of many shots. The end of a scene is typically marked by a change in location, style or time.

Scene, Master. See Master Scene.

Science Fiction. A film which is having accent on scientific elements.

Screen Techniques, Wide. The function of a theatre-screen is to reflect the illuminated image projected upon it, with the maximum efficiency, the minimum amount of colour distortion and the best possible distribution. RCA synchro-screen developed by Ben Schlenger has been recognised as one of the best wide screens methodically.

Screen Time. Time taken by a scene when it is projected on the screen is called the screen time of the screen.

Screening. An exhibition of a movie, typically at a cinema.

Screenplay. A film-script written to be filmed and produced as a movie.

Screenwriter. A film-writer who either adapts an existing work for production as a movie or creates a new screenplay.

Scribe. (In music). This instrument is used to scrape the emulsion from film to create a line (streamer).

Script. This is a general term for a written work detailing story, setting, and dialogue. A script may take the form of a screenplay, shooting/lined/continuity/spec script. A script is often sold by the owner for a particular price, which is increased to a second price if the script is produced as a movie.

Script Break-down Sheet. An important single document which refers to all the future references of the film production. The sheet consists of cast, extracts, atmosphere, silent bits, special props, vehicles, animals, wardrobe, makeup/Hair, sound effects/ music special equipment, production notes/etc. Estimated number of set-ups/production in time is written on Script Breakdown Sheets prepared by Production Manager and the same is prepared by him for each scene in the screenplay.

Script-bretwalda material. The basic material of the film-script. Any and every movement will not be able to build a film and hence basic material viz. movement will have to be selected. It must be selected for its significant. (Bretwalda is a title of certain kings of old English kingdoms, whose superiority over the others was always acknowledged during ancient period.)

Script Department. The section of a production's crew responsible for the script of a movie. Consists of writers, script editors and prompters.

Script Editing. (Script Editor/Doctor). A process whereby a script is reviewed and changed, based on input from various sources such as the Director or producer. The writers who specialized in script editing are called 'script doctors' and are frequently uncredited but well paid.

Script, Lined. See Lined Script.

Script, Running time of a. Though there is not any hard and fast rule. It is estimated at the rate of about one minute to the page typed on the right hand side (half portion) of a sheet in double space.

Script, Spec. See Spec Script.

Script Supervisor. A person who tracks which parts have been filmed and takes notes on all relevant details of each shots. He also makes a note as to how the filmed scenes deviated from the script. Script Supervisor also makes continuity notes creating a lined script. Formerly often called 'script girl'/'Continuity girl.

Seamstress. Seam is a line of junction between edges seen together or between other edges generally. Seamstress is a person who is engaged for making the costume of the scheduled film.

Second Unit. (2nd Unit). A small, subordinate crew responsible for filming shots of less importance such as insects, crowds, scenery etc.

Segue. (Particularly in Music). Smooth transition from one sound to another.

Sensitometry of Colour Material. Specialized developments of methods of black and white sensitometry.

Sequel. A movie that presents the continuation of characters and/or events of a previously filmed movie.

Sequence. This is a paragraph of a film. A related series of shots unified by some element they hold in common. Sequence is the major segment of a film.

Serial. A multi-part film that usually screened a chapter each week at a cinema. The story structure is usually having each chapter ending with a cliffhanger to ensure the audience would like to watch following chapter at its release.

Sequence of Lap Dissolve. See Lap Dissolve.

Series. (Franchise). A sequence of films with continuing characters or themes, but with little other interdependence, especially with respect to plot or significant character development.

Set. An environment-artificially constructed setting used for filming.

Set Decorator. (Set Decoration). A person in the team who has total charge of decorating the set with all furnishings, drapery, interior plants and anything seen on indoor or outdoor sets.

Set designer. The person responsible for translating a production designer' vision of the movie's environment into a set which can be used for filming.

Set Dresser. A person in the team who is responsible for the placement of all properties on the set in their proper positions and for the decoration of a set. A set dresser is also responsible for renting and/or purchasing all material that is needed to dress a set as required.

Set List. A list of all the settings to be used in the film.

Set Medic. This provides for the medical needs and emergency medical logistics of the entire cast and crew of the film production. It is the safety liaison between production/construction and various agencies.

Set, Plan and Elevation of. For planning and elevation of sets, an Art Director has to take into consideration several aspects. Due to the advancement of technique, state-of-art certain items from the following list have been deleted/replaced. But ordinarily Art Directors world-over prepare a big sheet of reminders for:

(i) Exterior wall surface: (a) Stone (b) Brick (c) Plaster (d) Wood.

(ii) Interior wall surface: (a) Patterned paper, (b) Plain paper, (c) Panelled, (d) Tapestry, (e) Moulding (f) Plaster.

(iii) Ceiling: (a) Plaster, (b) Canvas, (c) Felt.

(iv) Floor: (a) Planks, (b) Cobbles, (c) Stone, (d) Paper, (e) Painted Hassian.

(v) Painting: (a) Textures, (b) Colours, (c) Blowing.

(vi) Backings: (a) Painted, (b) Photographic, (c) Drapery.

(vii) Windows: (a) Practical, (b) Glass, (c) Exterior Wall and sill also water effects, smoke effects, other practicals, cobwebs curtains, illuminations etc.

Set up. Any particular camera position.

Setting. The physical surroundings in which a given segment of a film's action is supposed to transpire.

Seventh Art. The art of motion pictures. The term was coined in the year 1916 by Italian Poet and Pioneer Film Theoretician Mr. Ricciotto Canudo.

Shooting Script. The script from which a movie is made. This script usually contains numbered scenes and technical notes.

Short subject. (film). A film that is shorter than 60 minutes' duration. This term is in contrast with a feature film which is also called a full-length film.

Shooting Report. A record maintained for picture and sound during the shooting sessions.

Shooting Schedule. This is prepared in the form of production-board by the production department, as per the standard practice. The position is displayed on the movable board on production strips.

Shot. A continuous block of unedited footage from a single point of view. The basic unit of film structure.

Shot Composition. The arrangement of key elements within the frame.

Shot, Freek. Placing a camera so low to the ground that people, horses or trains seem to pass over it, or placing it so high above the head of the character so that the camera appears to shoot down upon them, as in top shot.

Shot List. Usually including slate numbers and an abbreviated discussions.

Shot, Martini. See Martini shot.

Shot Process. See Process Shot.

Shot Selection. (Camera Angle). The location of the camera, and what can be seen with it.

Shots, Assembling. Logically assembled shots by a consideration of the way in which an onlooker would use his eyes where he viewing the scene in real life.

Shoulder Shot. A shot taken from above the shoulder.

Shutter Speed. The length of time that a single frame is exposed for. Slower shutter speeds allow more light to enter the camera, but allow more motion blur.

Sibilance. Refers to the hiss created in speaking and recording of words that contain an emphatic 'S' sound which can result in problems.

Signal-to-Noise Ratio. The relationship between the specific sound require in a recording and the level of noise present in the background.

Silent Film. (Silent). A film that has no synchronized soundtrack and no spoken dialogue. It was a form predominate in films until the late 1920s when practical synchronization of sound technology was developed and its use became popular.

Silver Recovery Unit. A plant used for extracting all the silver that is regularly going into solution in a processing machine.

Single Stripe. A reel of 35 mm clear-base film with a narrow stripe of magnetic tape.

Situation. The Fictional circumstances prevailing as a film opens.

Situation comedy. (Sitcom) A comedy in which humour is derived from people being placed in uncomfortable, embarrassing on unfamiliar situations.

Sketch. Music with an indicated tempo and a melody line or theme written out.

Skin Flick. A sex film.

Skip Frame. Same as Fast Motion.

Slapstick Comedy. (Slapstick). A comedy in which the humour is derived from physical interactions, often involving exaggerated but ultimately harmless violence directed towards individuals. (This term has been named after a device used by circus clowns—two boards which slap together loudly when swatted on someone's backside).

Slate. The device process of denoting a shot during filming.

Slide Films. Series of 16 mm and 35 mm still picture arranged in sequences and projected frame by frame on screen. Sound slide films has narration on disc or tape which is cued to frames projected on screen.

Slow Motion. (Slow-Mo, Slow Mo). A shot in which time appears to move slowly than normal. The process is commonly achieved by either repeating frames or by over-cranking.

Slow Motion Process follows by slowing down of action in a scene caused by running the camera faster than the normal.

Slug Line. (Slug). A header appearing in the script before each scene or shot detailing the location, date and time that the following action is intended to occur in.

Sneak in. To bring in music or sound effects softy and then increase the volume.

Sneak preview. (Preview). An un-announced screening of the film before the premiere. This is very often used to gauge audience reaction and feedback for final editing.

Snow. For falling snow, very small feathers are some times used as they fly about very effectively when two or three small electric fans are placed around the set. For snow on the ground, marble dust is used and get glistening effect, Neptha is at times sprinkled on the top.

Snow Blindness. (In photography). Inflammation and painful sensitiveness to light caused by exposure of the eyes to ultraviolet rays reflected from snow or ice.

Society of Motion Picture and Television Engineers. (SMPTE). An international technical society devoted to advancing the theory and application of motion-imaging technology.

Society of Operating Cameraman. (SOC). US-based honorary organisation composed of several hundred men and women internationally, of outstanding and dedicated talent, who make their living operating film and/or video cameras in the cinematic media.

Soft Cut. A very short dissolve conveying the effect of a merging of two images but without implying passage of time or change of scene.

Soft Focus. Shooting subjects slightly out of focus to gain a lazy effect.

Songs. In most of the countries film songs play an important part. During silent era musical instruments were played as a background. For Lumieres' very first exhibition of films, a solo pianist was being engaged with the introduction of talkies very much importance was given to singing. Thus music has remained one of the striking features of films. In India, by and large the song and dance formula continued to dominate.

Sony Dynamic Digital Sound. (SDDS). Sony has produced a noise reduction and sound enhancement process. (Dolby Digital and DTS are the competitors).

Sound Characteristics of. Any sound contains frequency and volume. In sound film recording the frequency is obtained by changing the amount of light which strikes the film. The volume is represented by the magnitude of these changes.

Sound Crew. (Sound/Assistant/Engineer). The group of crew members directly involved with creating of a movie's sound track.

Sound Designer. The conceptual chief of a movie's soundtrack, responsible for designing and creating the audio component of a movie.

Sound Editor. A member of the sound crew who performs editing on the soundtrack.

Sound Effects. (SFX, FX). Sounds added during post-production by the sound crew. Also used as a job title.

Sound Effects Editor. A sound editor who specializes in editing sound effects.

Sound Film. Magnetic. See Magnetic Sound Film.

Sound Loop. A section of sound, usually of effects — that is joined head to tail for continuous running during mixing, normally for use as additional background sound when required.

Sound mix. (Mix). The process of re-recording multiple reels of track to produce one final soundtrack, which includes all dialogues. Looped dialogues (ADR), music, sound effects, foley, and narration.

Sound Mixer. An audio engineer who performs the sound mix.

Soundstage. A large area, usually in a studio, where elaborate sets may be constructed. Soundstages are preferred since they allow filmmakers greater control over factors such as sound, lighting temperature, spectators and security.

Soundtrack. Audio component of a movie. Popularly, it refers to a collection of songs which are heard during the movie, often sold as an album.

Soundtrack, Magnetic. See Magnetic Soundtrack.

Soundtrack, Optical. See Optical Soundtrack.

Sound Wave. Like light waves sound waves tell us about the conditions of things in the world in which we live, what these things ARE, and what at the moment they are doing. In such cases, we arrive without actual contact at a knowledge of these things across space, and actually at a much better and more thorough knowledge than is possible by the direct process or touch.

Source. Any medium like a junc box, muzak which can be a source of music.

Space Opera. A science fiction film.

Space Time Problem. It is complicated by six considerations: (i) Transition, (ii) Camera, (iii) Dialogue, (iv) Mobility of Narrative, (v) Audience contact, and (iv) Characteristic of Narrative.

Spacer. Blank leader of gash film that is used as such in building up sound tracks.

Spaghetti Wester. A western film filmed in Italy.

Speaking/Non-speaking Role. A speaking role is one in which the character speaks scripted dialogue. A non-speaking role is a character specifically mentioned in the script but who doesn't have any lines of dialogue in the finished film.

Spec Script. A script written before any agreement has been entered into on spec (speculation), in hopes of selling the script the highest bidder once it has been completed.

Special Effects. (SFX). An artificial effect used to create an illusion in a movie. This refers to effects produced on the set, as opposed to those created in post-production (visual effects).

Special Effects Supervisor. (Also Special Effects Co-ordinator) The chief of a production's special effects crew.

Special Make-up Effects. An artist who has expertise in combining makeup with special effects, producing squibs and other devices.

Speculation. Tendering film-script to producer on approval basis. In such cases, film-script writer gets his remuneration provided the producer accepts his script.

Speech, Clean. See Clean Speech.

Speed. This term refers to an announcement made by either the director of photography or camera operator indicating to the Director that the camera is operating at the correct speed. Speed is called just after lock it down and just before action.

Spherical/print. An optical system in which the magnifications of the vertical and horizontal dimensions of the picture are the same.

Spine. A film-script's basic plot.

Splice. The joining of two pieces of film by any of various techniques.

Splicer, Hot. See Hot Splicer.

Split Screen. Film so manipulated that different shots appear simultaneously in different sections of the screen when projected.

Spoken Titles. Dialogue rendered in the form of sub-titles.

Spotting Notes. In Music, any notes made after the spotting session.

Sprocket Holes. Holes along both sides of 35 mm film. These are, however, on only one side of 16 mm films.

Squib. A small explosive device which when detonated, will simulate the effect of a bullet/puncture wound or small explosion. When worn by actors, they typically include a container of blood which bursts upon detonation.

Stand in. (Also Stand-in). A person who has the same physical properties of a particular actor and takes their place during the lengthy set up of a scene. This allows the actor to prepare for the filming itself. The term 'squib' is in contrast with stunt/body double.

Standby Painter. A scenic artist available during filming for the last minutes changes/touches.

Star. (Screen Star). A celebrated actor or/and actress.

Start Frame. Any agreed-on frame to set a footage or seconds counter at zero.

Start Marks. These are put in—films in with wax pencil to indicate where picture and sound films are to be placed in the moviola or inter-lock projector to be in sync.

Static. Marks caused by a discharge of static electricity during the photographic process.

Steadicam. A camera attached to a camera operator via a mechanical harness which reduces or eliminates the unsteadiness of the operator's motion. A camera operator who operates steadicam is called a Steadicam Operator. In United States Steadicam Operators Association (SOA) has been established world-over. Steadicam operators providing the facility across the entire film and video industry are the members of SOA.

Stem. In sound recording of one of the magnetic recording track areas on the dubbed master track.

Step outline. A sequence outline of a feature on a television film, specifying action to take place as a story goes on developing.

Stills Photographer. A person in the team who photographs the film actions often alongside the camera. These stills are mostly used in publicizing the movie.

Sting. A striking sound which is used as emphasis of punctuation in a film.

Stock. Film stock, the celluloid compound itself before exposure.

Stock Footage. For the various reasons like simplicity, time or a budget, some shots in a film are duplicated from other films or a film library. These are called 'Stock footage' of duly filmed shots drawn from the film libraries to eliminate the need for shooting the sequence involved.

Stooges. The Three. Comedy team specializing in violent, vulgar slapstik. Approximately 200 Three stooges shorts were produced by Columbia between the years 1934 and 1958.

Stop Motion. (Stop-Motion). A form of animation in which objects are filmed frame-by-frame and slightly in between each frame.

Story Analyst. A studio story department employee who appraises and synopsizes potential screen play material.

Story Construction. As far as the structure of the story is concerned it may be divided into three parts viz. the dramatic form/play form, fiction form/literary form and synopsis form/Composite form.

Story Factors. Since utmost care has to be taken to see that audiences attention does not wander for an instant, three prime factors in the construction of a film story are always taken into considerations. These are balance, timing and economy.

Story, Phases of. There are 3 phases of a story or a plot. (1) The premise, (2) The complications, and (3) The resolution. In terms of time the exposition of premise is about one sixth the playing time of a picture or television programmes. Two third is given to the various complications and one sixth to the resolution of the story. The complication is the main body of a picture or television programme.

Story, Speed of the. Basically there are three recognised speeds of the story viz. Rapid Moderate and Leisurely.

Story Telling Systems. These are two systems of film story telling. Straight forward and Flash back.

Story, Timing of. The introduction, at precisely the right moment of the different elements of the story.

Storyboard. A sequence of pictures created by a production illustrator to communicate the desired general visual appearance on camera of a scene or movie.

Straight cut. Used for differentiate the normal joining together of shots from those involving optical effects.

Streamer. In music a visual line moving from one side of a screen.

Stripe Edge. See Edge strip.

Studio. A company that makes films.

Stunt. (Gag). A non-trivial and often dangerous piece of physical action. Very often performed by a stunt performer.

Stunt Co-ordinator. A person in a team who arranges and plans stunts for film shooting.

Stunt Double. A stunt performer who specifically takes the part of another actor for a stunt.

Stunt Performer. (Stunt Player/Stunts). A/specialist actor who performs stunts.

Stylist. Contributor to the look of a movie by choice.

Stylus. Of clothes, decor or other items of fashion.

In music, an instrument used to scrape a narrow line in a piece of film.

Subjective Camera. A technique sometimes used in instrumental films in which the camera approximates the learner's point of view.

Sub-Plot. A story within a story.

Sub-Standard. Sizes of film stock smaller than that is used in commercial cinemas which is 35 mm is known as sub-standard film. There are 3 sub-standard sizes viz. 16 mm, 9.5 mm and 8 mm. Sub-standard stock differs from 35 mm, in that it is non-inflammable.

Sub-titles. Most often subtitles are in different language than that which is being spoken. But sometimes for different reasons sub-titles are also given for the film in the same language the spoken words are applied. For example, in 'Trainspotting' (1966) subtitles were used for getting humorous effect. Sub-titles are given in the process of superimposing the words heard on the screen.

Subtractive method. Before the 3-colour process TECHNICOLOR presented a 2-colour process where the two negatives were being obtained by means of a beam-splitting camera. In this process the resultant dye images were being cemented back to back.

Subtractive Printing. When printing is done in the ordinary white light and all correction, i.e. addition of a tinge of one colour or the other, is done by introducing filters in the path of the printing beam of light, supplementary in colour to the colour of the desired correction, it is called a subtractive printing.

Suspense. It has been said that the suspense is the secret of mobility and the foundation of suspense is motive. Surprise should be as a substitute for suspense. Average distance between these points of suspense in the story, according to the experts, should run into 700 to 800 feet. Uncertainty of outcome, the fear that something will or will not happen.

Sustaining 'Super -16' Method. A method of photographic on 16 mm film using a camera with a special gate plate, to produce a wide screen format. This is for blowing up on to 35 mm film. In India quite a few low-budget films' producers have experimented in this method. But filmgoers have on the whole not accepted such films. Super-16 format allows 40 per cent more exposable frame area to film-makers.

Swimming. (In music). Instrumental sounds moving within the orchestra and distorting clear resolution.

Sword and Sorcery. A colloquialism for genre of film, usually set in days of old with magic as well as sword fighting.

Sync. License. License permitted by a film song's publisher to use by charging fees.

Sync Pulse. Any electronic pulsation that is recorded on tape and used to control speed.

Sync Sound. Usually dialogue recorded at the time of production shoot.

Synchronization. Exact matching of a film's sound and action, as of speech and lip movements.

Synchronous Sound. Sound recorded at the same time as picture, with camera and recorder linked together.

Synopsis. A summary of a major plot points and characters of a script, generally in a page or two. The term is in contrast with treatment.

Synthesis. The combination of separate elements of thought into a whole for example In 'East Meets West' (musical album) synthesis, celebrated violinist Yehudi Menuhin and Sitar Mastero Pt. Ravi Shankar have made a whole out of parts from both Eastern and Western music.

T

Tag Line. (Curtain/Punch Line). The final speech in a confrontation, episode or sequence.

Tail-away shot. Movement directly away from the camera, as and when a shot is of the back of a man departing.

Take. A single continuous recorded performance of a scene.

Talent. A general informal term for actors and also for extras.

Talkies, First Line in. Al Jolson's 'The Jazz Singer (1927) is the very first publicly performed sound film in the history of world talkies. The first line of 'The Jazz Singer' was "Wait a minute, wait a minute, you ain't heard nothing yet! Wait a minute, I tell you. You ain't heard nothing yet! Do you want to hear? Toot, Toot, Tootsie?"

Talkies, First Premiere of. United Kingdom's premiere of 'The Jazz Singer' took place on September 27, 1928 at Piccadilly Theatre. However this film was first shown at the Warner Theatre in New York, America on October 6, 1927.

Tape Recorder Operator. (Sound Recordist). A member of the sound crew responsible for operating the audio recording equipment on a set.

Tape Splicer. An apparatus to cut and join film together using transparent adhesive tape.

Target Audience. A group to which a film is designed to appeal.

Teaser. Especially in a television picture intriguing pre-title action used to capture audience attention.

Technical Advisor. (Consultant). A person with expertise in a particular field who provides advice for the production.

Technicolour. The first technicolour laboratory was built within a railway car at Boston. In 1917 this car was transported to Florida for the first technicolour film entitled 'The Gulf Between'.

Teleplay. A script written to be produced for television.

Television Cut-off. The area of the frame that is actually visible in the television transmission.

Television Movie. (TV Movie, Telepic). A feature length movie funded by a TV network, intended to the premiered on television.

Television Special. A television production of a singular event such as an awards show or concert, as opposed to a regularly scheduled series. This is in contrast with series and television movie.

Telewriter. A writer who either adapts an existing work in different forms for production of television, or creates a new teleplay.

Tempo. An impression of pace in film. Also (in music) number of beats per minute.

Theatre system, Digital. See Digital Theatre Systems.

Theme. A screen play implicit message.

Third World Cinema. The term applies to films made in countries which have been in the primary stages, unable to sustain an individual film culture because of poverty, domination by foreign powers or political oppression.

THX (The THX Division). A sub-division of Lucasfilm Ltd. dedicated to improving picture and sound for the cinema and the home.

Tilt. The action of rotating the either up or down during the taking of a shot.

Time Code. A visually displayed or hidden group.

Time Lapse Photography. (Time Lapse). A form of animation in which numerous single frames are filmed spaced at a given interval to show a process that would take a very long time to occur. Flower blooming and motion of the stars are the examples of time lapse form.

Timer. A laboratory specialist.

Timing. In music description of actions and dialogue noted by seconds and tenth of seconds on the music breakdown sheets.

Title Design. (Title Designer/Sequence, Titles). The manner in which title of a film is displayed on screen is widely considered as an art form. Saul Bass — US Graphic Designer — is considered a master title. Bass is best known for the black alley cat credit sequence in 'Walk on the Wild Side' (1962) which, like all his best work, brilliantly and economically establishes the predominant theme of the film.

Title, Spoken. See Spoken Title.

TMT Technique. The Ten Minutes Take (TMT) technique was introduced by Alfred Hitchock. In this system one single shot is taken continuously without breakings for ten minutes.

Titra. A patented process where the emulsion is removed from the film to produce the subtitles.

Tone. A film-makers treatment of subject matter designed to produce a specific audience responses.

Track. A single component or channel of a soundtrack. To move the camera bodily forward or backward during the taking of a shot.

Track, International. See International Track.

Tracking Shot. (Tracking). The action of moving a camera along a path parallel to the path of the object being filmed.

Tracklaying. In film editing, the process of assembling sound film of all kinds in a form that allows for efficient manipulation during mixing.

Tracks. Dolly. See Dolly Tracks.

Trailer. An ad for a movie which contains sporadic scenes from the film. Formerly these ads were attached to the end of the newsreel. Also blank film at the end of a reel after the last shot.

Transfer, Dye. See 'Dye Transfer'.

Transition. The bridge from one confrontation to another.

Transportation Co-ordinator/Manager. A person in the team responsible for managing transport section.

Travelling Matte Shot. (Blue Screen). A shot in which foreground action is superimposed on a separately filmed background by optical printing or digital compositing.

Treatment. An abridged script which is longer than a synopsis. While a complete script is around 100 pages, a treatment of the same is of 10 to 12 pages.

Trim. A short section of any shot or sound track that has been removed from the take as assembled or cut into the film.

Trim Bin. The device in which trims are hung or clipped while the materials for a sequence is being cut.

Trucking Shot. Dolly shot.

Tungsten Halogen Light. An incandescent lamp with long life, constant colour temperature and virtual freedom from blackening. Also see Quartz lights.

Two Shot. A shot taken so as to include two people only in a frame with their head and shoulders.

U

Ultrasonic. A method of cleaning dirt from film by use of high frequency sound waves.

Undercranking. The process of slowing down the frame rate of a camera down so that when the captured pictures are played at the normal frame rate the action appears to be in fast motion.

Underground Film. A term originating in the United States in the late 1950s and applied to the area of film-making hitherto described as experimental, personal, independent and/or avant-garde.

Underscore. Music designed for the emotional enhancement of a production.

Undershot. A sequence or a whole film inadequately covered in the shooting which makes film-editing unnecessary difficult.

Unit Production Manager. (UMP also Unit Manager). An executive who is responsible to a senior producer for the administration of a particular film.

UP. Increased volume of music or sound effects.

Utiliscope. A closed-circuit television system developed by Diamond Power Speciality Corporation, Lancaster. Simplicity in circuits and controls is a basic feature of utiliscope.

V

Values of the picture. (i) Cost (ii) Star values (iii) Fashion values (iv) Director values (v) Music values (vi) Story values (vii) Market values.

Varioscope. A device introduced by architect Ben Schelenger which enables the constant changing of the aspect ratio on a given screen area without changing lenses or aperture plates in film projection.

Versatile Disc, Digital. See Digital versatile disc.

Versions, Foreign. Before acquiring the success in dubbing process, film producers were bringing out foreign versions of their films to enable them to obtain international market for their films. America and Germany were the prominent producers of such versions.

Video. The side of the two column script describing the action to the filmed (the visual on the left side).

Video Cassette Recorder. (VCR) A common household appliance for recording and/or playing pre-recorded video tapes.

Video Disc. A disc similar to the gramophone record on which information is stored in digital form and is used to record television picture, as a computer memory unit etc.

Video Home System. (VHS) is a popular format for VCR systems world-wide.

Video Parlour. (Also known as Video Mini Theatre). Since 1985, numerous Indian entrepreneurs have established the video parlours as one of their small-scale industries. It has already been recognised as 'industry' by different state governments. As per Maharashtra Cinema (Regulations) Amended Act, 1987, all the video parlours exhibiting cinema on video have to obtain licenses from the proper authorities. At present approximately 2200 video parlours are exhibiting their shows in Maharashtra.

Viewer. A mechanical/optical enlarging unit used by film-editors to examine the film.

Virgin Loops. Mint sound film that is looped for the purposes of recording especially during post-synchronisation.

Vista-vision. A photographic process introduced by Paramount Pictures which claimed that the best print and in turn the best large screen picture is witnessed through this process.

Visual Effects. Alterations to a film's images during post-production.

Visual Field. The entire expanse of space visible at a given instant without moving the eyes.

Voice Over. (V). Indicates that the dialogue will be heard on a movie's soundtrack, but the speaker will not be shown.

Voltameter. An instrument for measuring in volts the difference of potential between different points of an electric circuit.

Volume. Fullness or quantify of tone.

W

Walla. (Also 'Rhubarb). Background conversation. Historically, when a script called for 'crowd unrest' or 'murmuring', the extras would be required to mumble the word 'rhubarb', as this produced the required effect.

Wardrobe Supervisor. See Costume Designer/Supervisor.

Warm Colours. Trombones, cellos, or midranged woodwings played with feeling are referred to as warm colours in musical orchestrations. (High violin section, tense with no vibrato depict cold colours.

Waveform monitor. An electronic scope used to measure and adjust various elements of a video signal. The waveform is used primarily to ensure consistency of the luminance (light intensity) of a video picture.

Weekend Opening. See Opening Weekend.

Weenie. An objectionification of the hero's desire in simplistic/not so simplistic films.

Westar VI. A satellite was previously known as 'Westar VI'. This was initially constructed in India by the Hughes Aircraft Company for Western Union — ASIASAT.

Western. (Oater/Oat Opera). A movie set in the 'Wild West' of the pre-civil was United States.

Western, Spaghetti. See Spaghetti Western.

Western Opening Weekend. See 'Opening Weekend.'

Whip Pan. (Whip-Pan). An extremely fast pan incorporating much motion blur. The term refers to the 'whipping action that the camera operator uses to move the camera.

Whip Over. Special use of too quick pan.

Wide Angle. A lens embracing an angle of view that is wider than usual.

Widescreen. A movie which has an aspect ratio which is greater than academy ratio when projected.

Wild. Film shot or sound recorded with no synchronous relationship with each other.

Wild Line. A line of dialogue with no visible sync.

Wild Sound. This is also called Mit Out Sound (MOS). Scenes that are filmed without the sound being recorded at the same time.

Wind Creating. In films, wind is created by mounting giant fans that agitate 8,000 cubic feet of air per minute on the moveable trollies.

Winners of Oscar Awards. Categories of Annual Oscar Awards are presented for the excellence in the following film categories. The venue of the events till recent days is Los Angeles' Shrine Auditorium. Film Categories: Best Director, Best Actor, Back-to-back Actor, Best Actress, Supporting Actor, Supporting Actress, Foreign Language Film, Original Screenplay, Screenplay Adaptation, Cinematography, Film Editing, Sound, Sound Effects Editing, Art Direction, Visual Effects, Costume, Design, Makeup, Song, Original Score, Documentary, Short Subject, Documentary Feature, Live Action Short Film, Animated Short Film, Jean Hersholt Humanitarian Award, Irving Thalberg Memorial Award and Honorary Award.

WipAn editing technique in which images from one shot are fully replaced by the images of another, delimited by a definite border that moves across or around the frame.

Word-of-mouth. Communication. This is via the spoken word on a person-to-person basis. Movie goers can't help warning their friends whether or not they should see that particular film about which a frank opinion is expressed by a person who saw it earlier. Gradually this opinion expressed by the first viewer can make or mar the business in the longer run.

Work Picture. The first colour print of a film used by the film editor. The negative is cut to match the picture.

Work Print. The positive copy of the print. This copy of film footage is used in editing so that the original will not be damaged.

Working Title. The name by which a movie is known while it is being made. This is sometime different from the title with which it is.

World Wide Web. (WWW). The faster growing part of the internate (internet). Many web pages are multimedia, although the disadvantage is that they then become slow to download.

WoW. A disturbance in sound that gives the effect of spasmodic changes etc.

Wrangler. (Also Animal Handler). A person in the team who is responsible for the care and control of entities used on a set that cannot be spoken with. This person is typically a professional consultant with expertise in handling the item, often with expertise in handling the item of a movie set. Wrangler is involved in the work of handling of live stock everything from mules to mosquitoes.

Wrap. (Windup, Wind). To finish shooting, either for the day or the entire production. A concluded sequence.

Writer. A general term for someone who creates a written work, be it a novel, script, screen-play or teleplay.

Writer's Guild of America. (WGA). This is the sole collective bargaining representative for writers in the motion picture, cable, broadcast, interactive and new media industries. The Guild is affiliated to numerous national and international writing organisations.

X

X Certificate. British Board of Film Censors (BBFC) introduced this category to designate films unsuitable for children.

Xenophonia. Reflection of tone.

XXX. An information voluntary certificate for a pornographic film. It indicates large amount of explicit sex covered in the film.

Xylonite. Cinema film. Celluloid. Non-thermosetting plastic of the nitrocellulose type.

Xylophone. A musical instrument consisting of a graduate series of wooden bars, which are rested on straw etc. and are struck by wooden hammers.

Y

Yankee Peddlers. Representatives of Lumiere Brothers—French inventors and pioneers of cinema are described as 'Yankee Peddlers. The original Yankee Peddlers were based in New England and are considered the forerunner of the modern day travelling salesperson.

Yarn. A slang for anapocryphal story.

Yell. Organised cry of spectators encouraging film personalities in celebrating events.

Yodel/Yodle. (In film music). To sing or shout, changing frequently from the ordinary voice to false to and back again after the manner of the mountaineers of the Tirol. In Indian (Hindi/Marathi) film music an actor and singer Kishore Kumar introduced yodelling. It has not been possible to any other singer till the turn of the century to imitate him in this respect.

Z

Zero Frame. The first frame of a roll of picture.

Zoetrop. Optical toy in the form of cylinder with series of pictures on inner surface which give impression of continuous motion when viewed through slits with cylinder rotating. The application of photography to the Zoetrope on 'When of Life' was first made about 1880 by Pritchard.

Zoom Lens. A lens with the variable focal length.

Zoom Shot. A shot in which the magnification of the objects by the camera's lenses is increased (zoom in) or decreased (zoom out/back). Alfred Hitchcock's much-imitated shot in 'Vertigo' (1958) used a combination zoom in and dolly resulting in a dramatic change in perspective.

Zoopraziscope. Modification of Zoetrope made by Edward J. Muybridge which enables projecting the glass plate on a screen.

Zorro Films. Originally inspired by the novel entitled 'The Curse of Capistrano' by Johnston McCulley numerous films based on the legendary masked-man adventures have been filmed. Zorro —a swash buckling character has been made popular by Douglas Fairbanks (Sr) and Tyrone Power. In 1981 George Hamilton appeared as Zorro in the film "Zorro, The Gay Blade."

Bibliography

A list of selected film–books in the English language

Anderson, L,:	Making a Film
Arnheim R.:	Film as Art
Bawden, Anne (ed.):	The Oxford Companion to Film.
Bazin, Andre et al:	What is Cinema?
Bjorkman Stig et al:	Bergman on Bergman.
Bresson R.:	Notes on Cinematography
Briley, John:	Gandhi (The screen-play).
Carrick F:	Designing for Films.
Corliss, Richard (ed):	The Hollywood Screenwriters.
Fisenstein, Sergie:	Film Form & Film Sense.
Geduld, Harry:	Film makers on Film making.
Graham, Peter:	The Dictionary of Cinema.
Graham, P:	The New Wave.
Griffith, Richard & Mayer Arthur:	The Movies.
Haliwell, L:	The Filmgoers Companion.

Jacobs, Lewis: The Movies as Medium.

Jacobs, L.: Introduction to the Art of Movies.

Katz, Ephraim: The Film Encyclopaedia.

Kaufamann, S & Henstall, B: American Film Criticism.

Knight, Arthur: The Liveliest Apt.

Manwell, Roger (Ed.): The International Encyclopaedia of Film.

O'brien, Geoffrey: The Phantom Empire.

Quigley, M: New Screen Technique.

Ray, Satyajit: My Years with Apu.

Robins, David: World Cinema.

Rotha, Paul: Documentary Film.

Sarrism, Andrew (ed): Interviews with Film Directors.

Saton, Maria: Portrait of a Director: Satyajit Ray.

Schickel, M. Matinee Idylls: Reflection on the Movies.

Spottishwood, R.: Film & Its Techniques.

Spottishwood, R.: Grammar of Film.

Thompson K & Bordwell, D: Film History: An Introduction.

Vardac, A. Nicholas: Stage to Screen

Wheeler A: Principles of Cinematography.

Besides the above publications, numerous books on films & filming published by Focal Press, and special monograms brought out by Institutions and organizations devoted to films and filming.